Praise for

NEW MOTHER

If you are pregnant or are a new mother you cannot afford not to heed the advice given by Allie Chee in her book, **New Mother,** *if you want to experience the true joy and fulfillment of new motherhood.
A very practical book written with humor and wisdom.*

DR. MAO SHING NI, PH.D., D.O.M., DIPL. ABAAHP

New Mother *is the book that should be in the hands of every woman with childbearing on her mind. Jam-packed with great information...* **New Mother** *dishes out practical advice in a fun and accessible way. Want to have a baby and live to tell about it? Get this book... and heed the advice!*

– CHRISTINA PIRELLO

Emmy award-winning host of the National Public Television series, 'Christina Cooks';

Author of 7 bestselling cookbooks, including *Cooking the Whole Foods Way*

New Mother *combines practical and helpful information from Eastern and Western practices for pregnancy and postpartum. I will recommend it to my patients and students.*

-DR. NING X. FU, O.M.D., PH.D

Professor, Five Branches University of Traditional Chinese Medicine

Allie Chee's new book provides the perfect antidote for a society that needs to shift its emphasis away from the superwoman image—towards a new and healthier philosophy that honors and nurtures one's body in a gentle and beautiful way.

This gem of a book details important information for moms-to-be and should be required reading provided by every midwife's and OB-GYN's practice.

-JOY FELDMAN, NC, JD

Author of *Joyful Cooking in the Pursuit of Good Health* and *Is Your Hair Made of Donuts?*

Allie may technically be a stranger, but she's your new best friend. Although motherhood is biological, it is also culturally generated, and this guide fits our time and place. Delight in the support you will feel by reading this book.

– HARRIET BEINFIELD, L.Ac.

Co-author, *Between Heaven and Earth: A Guide to Chinese Medicine*

The book for all expectant moms... and dads... to really understand WHY they need help when they have a new baby!

It is not about being able to do it yourself. It is about getting the support that you need and empowering you in your new role. Excellently and especially written for women who are passionate about helping families!

– CHRISTINE GOLDMAN, CD, CPD, CBE, LE

NEW MOTHER

New Mother

Using a Doula, Midwife, Postpartum Doula, Maid, Cook, or Nanny to Support Healing, Bonding, and Growth

Allie Chee

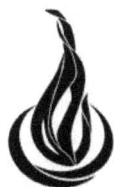

HESTIA
BOOKS & MEDIA

Published in the United States by
Hestia Books & Media
1111 West El Camino Real, #109-207
Sunnyvale, CA 94087

ISBN-13: 978-0-9856264-0-2

Library of Congress Control Number: 2012909521

First Hestia Books & Media edition 2012.

Cover design by Laura Coyle
Interior illustrations by Jillian Dister
Book design and layout by LUCITÀ Inc.

Visit http://www.alliechee.com for more information about Allie Chee and her work.

Printed in the United States of America on FSC-certified, 30% post consumer recycled paper.

Dedication

To Babies

We long for them.

We pray for them.

We wait months, years, and sometimes decades for them.

We save every penny for them.

We plan all we will do, be, and give to them.

We wait for the "perfect time" and make sacrifices along the way for them.

And when we are blessed with them, they have only one desire… to be with us.

So let's BE with our babies!

DEDICATION

To Parents

This book is written for parents who want to be with their children.

It may seem obvious that all parents would want to be with their baby, so what does that mean?

Many mothers want to have the full, natural experience of their pregnancy and childbirth, but they are unfamiliar with the process, too full of fears. So they concede to a template experience.

Many mothers would like to rest and spend beautiful time bonding with their babies immediately after birth and for several months postpartum, but they don't know how, and they don't know that it's natural and expected all around the world. What's worse, many don't think they can afford to (although, fortunately, they usually can). They don't even know what they don't know, so they accept a compromised experience.

Many parents hire help or put their children in daycare because they are overwhelmed, exhausted, and pressured—internally or externally—about getting back to a "regular" life and back to work. This leaves less time to spend with their children.

This book is written for people who want to find a way to be with their babies as much as possible, day and night—without turning into zombies. It is for people with high standards who are looking for more time with their babies, for those who want to feed, teach, and entertain them. It's for parents who want to just BE with them as much as possible—even if they feel too tired to read this book.

Though that's not what we're told, taught, or empowered to do, it is possible to have it all: a more natural experience; fun, relaxing family time; time to care for the house; time to care for yourself; the power to choose whatever vision you hold for your birthing and motherhood experience.

Contents

ACKNOWLEDGMENTS

With Special Thanks To . . .

My mother, who held the family together against the odds.

Turkan Yukselen, for showing me the beauty and joy in homemaking.

Tony Braubach, for introducing me, at age 10, to the concept of "you are what you eat," and for his continued friendship to this day.

My husband, Meng, who shared my vision of family life with father as the primary provider and mother as the full-time homemaker.

For help with this book: my editors David Colin Carr and Birgitte Rasine; Birgitte's company LUCITÀ for book design; my cover designer Laura Coyle; and my illustrator Jillian Dister.

And above all, my daughter Celestine, and all babies, for being our greatest teachers and the lights of our lives.

INTRODUCTION

My Journey to Motherhood and Why I Offer This to You

'd always imagined a natural birth. In our twenties my cousin Christina and I joked about squatting in the shade of a tree to have our babies. We were just joking—but not completely.

Throughout my thirties I watched not one or two, but almost all my friends enthusiastically enter the hospital in labor, having claimed for nine months that they would have a natural birth. Yet they came out two (or ten) days later having been induced, forced to labor on their back, drugged, cut, and observed by countless strangers. Their babies had been taken from them immediately after birth and they were having nursing problems.

If you'd asked them ahead of time if that would have been their story, none of them would have said yes. These were fit, health conscious women. I wondered what had gone on behind the doors of the L&D that all of them were checking out with dramatically altered birth stories.

In my third trimester I attended an all-day birthing class at a store for "new moms" and babies. The store had been an excellent resource for me—I found great products there and particularly enjoyed their book and DVD library—so I was looking forward to the class.

The women in attendance were from around the world, highly educated in their fields of work, and well to do with all conveniences of life available to them.

And yet... here are some things I heard during class:

- "I've heard that babies nurse every two hours when they are born, but that won't work because I sleep about nine or so hours per night. What will happen to my breast milk during the nine hours that I'm sleeping?" (after telling the class that her father was an OB-GYN).

- "I've never heard of a birth without an epidural... I didn't know it was possible." This one looked like a presidential candidate, in an immaculate navy blue suit, pearls, and perfect shoulder-length hair and manicured nails.

- "I just want to go back to work as soon as possible, but I'll feel like a cow pumping—I can't do it" (spoken through tears).

- "What is the areola?" asked on learning how to help the

baby latch. She was surprised to hear that a part or all of it could be in the baby's mouth while he nursed.

• That weaning the baby from the breast 7-9 times a day was something you decided one day and switched to formula or cow's milk in bottles the next.

• That one minute the water breaks and immediately afterward the baby makes her exit.

• Most of the women had not heard of meconium, nor why it's important to know about.

• Most hadn't heard of swaddling and none of us knew how to swaddle a baby properly.

• Not one had considered a homebirth.

• Not one had considered a natural birth.

• We were all concerned about the increasing contractions in our third trimester, though they are normal as the uterus preps for the big day.

• "How much is it going to hurt?" and "How can I avoid the pain?" were the primary concerns of almost all in attendance.

Although I had already studied so much, explored, and found quality help, I attended the class to learn more about childbirth and postpartum care of baby and mom. But these women were only now seeking education and help.

What they received, though, was a lecture about towing the industry line:

- You will have an epidural and likely other drugs.

- There's a high chance that you'll have a C-section (and here's a video so you can see what it looks like).

- Postpartum instruction: if you are going to drink wine, pump first—if you breastfeed—or "pump and dump" after you drink.

Women were being trained to think of childbirth and postpartum as a "procedure"—to be endured and gotten through as quickly and painlessly as possible—and to rely entirely on a system that was treating them as a "workforce" and "profit center" rather than a family being gifted with another spirit in their lives.

There was no focus on natural childbirth. No mention of home birth (except when they asked everyone which hospital they were using, and I said I was having my baby at home). No discussion of postpartum as a healing, bonding, growing, significant, and once-in-a-lifetime experience for mother, father, and baby.

A treasure lost for those parents and babies. Precious, fleeting time and experiences that will never come again!

The lecturing nurse approached me during the break and said, "I'm really happy you're here today. It's nice to engage with someone who takes this seriously and can stand firmly on the ground of the decisions they've made about birth and motherhood."

I asked her why she was focusing on a grim, mechanical approach to childbirth.

To her credit, she accepted my question and said, "I'd like to cover other material, but it always seems that this is the information the mothers want."

I wasn't sure about that, but I was listening.

I asked her if this level of ignorance about birth and babies in third-trimester moms was always so high, or if this group was a fluke collection of the most uninformed and misguided women on Earth.

She said it is always like this, that mothers only care about avoiding pain.

I had a different vision for my childbirth and postpartum experience, and I believe if those women and thousands—if not millions—of other expecting moms knew of other options, if they knew they could get natural, loving, nurturing help, they would create a different vision for their own childbirth and postpartum time.

Over the weeks and months of my pregnancy, about once a day I heard, "Wow, you must write about this. I've never heard of *anyone* doing *that!*" (whatever we were talking about at the moment).

We're not just talking about any ol' person I bumped into at the gas station. I heard it from American mothers, Chinese grandmothers, people from all over the world, from my midwives, and even from my OB-GYN. Enough generations of women have lived under the current norms—even in places with ancient traditions—that the more natural and should-be-obvious ways have been almost completely forgotten or are considered too difficult.

Taking the Road Less Traveled

Do we all need to deliver at home with a midwife, stay home with our babies, nurse for two years, use cloth diapers, co-sleep, prepare three home-cooked organic meals a day, and have the support of a postpartum doula as well as domestic help?

That's not for everyone—but it's what I wanted.

My background offered no ideas or experience for how to do it, so I fully empathize with those women from the birthing class!

I grew up in Texas as a latchkey kid of a hard working, almost-broke mother who had smarts and tenacity, but no loving family background or experience of her own to guide her. My absentee alcoholic father—the handful of times he did show up—well, at least he was sweet and fun, if not sober. I was born in a hospital with my mother unconscious (they called it "a block" back then). I was then taken to a plastic box where a bunch of other babies were alone, cold, and crying in their separate plastic boxes, and I was bottle-fed formula.

We're not talking *Little House on the Prairie* here.

And my mother's postpartum time? Aunties and grandmothers to help her? Maybe a neighbor or two? Nah, they weren't really help. They were what many women in those roles are today—essentially a "friend" who comes to visit from time to time and sometimes shows up with a greeting card and store-bought blanket made of plastic materials or a take-out dinner.

They were certainly not the grandmothers or aunties of other times and places who doted on a new mother and baby, cooked, cleaned, knitted blankets and booties, guided (yes, sometimes too much), and supported in a thousand spontaneous ways.

So my poor mother did her best, barely surviving the cold, mechanical system.

Like her, many women today struggle through the modern "process," completely unaware that it could be another way, not knowing how to improve on the situation even if they wanted to.

Other women go through the experience feeling that all that was sacred and beautiful about pregnancy and motherhood had been compromised, wanting more, but not knowing how to make it better.

Yet some figure out how to do it a different way.

How did I come to my path?

Lots and lots and lots of reading, watching DVDs, attending classes, grilling doctors, interviewing midwives, hunting for mothers who had a different approach, living all over the world, anthropological research, questioning the information I found and things people said. And sitting still and asking myself: *what feels right?*

After all the preparing, planning, and praying, deciding on an all-natural pregnancy, home birth, and postpartum time came down to just a few things for me: faith that my baby and my body would know what to do; and the by-God-I-can-pick-up-this-bus grit to do it, despite so many sources saying I shouldn't and not seeing many others doing it.

What does it take to develop that level of faith and grit? Different things for different women. I can tell you what I did.

Long before I conceived, I had been living a unique lifestyle in preparation for conception, pregnancy, and motherhood. I had refined my diet, activities, and environment—even my thoughts and words—to support my intention to live in health, gratitude, and love. I traveled and studied extensively, and through these experiences around the world I was introduced to Traditional Chinese Medicine (TCM) and Ayurveda.[1]

---

1. My ongoing study of health and nutrition initiated changes. Between twenty to forty, I went from a diet comprised exclusively of processed and fast foods to a diet comprised exclusively of organic, home made, whole foods. The pursuit began with a typical Western approach to nutrition: less soda and pizza, more fruit and more veggies, and lots of juicing—wheat grass juice was the rage. The next phase was experimenting with a vegetarian diet

During pregnancy I found almost all my answers in those ancient systems. Where there were gaps, I dug elsewhere and asked for help from my loving midwives, doctors, and doulas.

When faced with those thousand questions that pop into a pregnant woman's mind at 2:00 in the morning, I turned to that place where people turn today for all aspects of family life, including recipes, groceries, directions for removing stains, tips on knitting and investing, spiritual guidance, friendship, and even true love:

The Internet.

I had the natural conception, pregnancy, home birth, and traditional 40-day postpartum that I dreamed of for my baby and myself at home—with wonderful help. The experiences were the most intensely beautiful moments of my life. But getting there wasn't easy. I went through several OB-GYNs, rightfully suspecting that they encouraged unnecessary interventions for insurance issues or convenience.

I went through a few midwives, not "feeling it" with the first two of them either.

---

and then vegan. The pursuit evolved to the study of Eastern food and health philosophies, which I found to be more balanced complete systems. For my goals and lifestyle, TCM and Ayurveda were the two systems that offered the best approach to radiant health and longevity. While I still study nutrition and health, the focus remains in TCM and Ayurveda. They are so rich and deep in ancient knowledge; one could study them for a lifetime and learn something fascinating and valuable every day.

I already had a highly trusted Traditional Chinese Medicine doctor.

I went through dozens if not hundreds of books, websites, and blogs, looking for knowledge to make the decisions about how to have my baby.

It was not "right decisions" I was looking for—but decisions about making the experience safe, relaxed, and *sacred*.

It was my body and my baby, after all. That was my responsibility, with help from many others of course. I could never accept a ready-made, drive-through-window solution served up by industries.

In this journey of discovery, I encountered many professionals who were telling mothers what to do, though they had never themselves had a baby (the gents obviously, but ladies too). Most people take that for granted today and never question their doctor's lack of experience.

Let's say that again: many women's primary or exclusive source of information and care are from people without personal experience, however many years in practice they have. Those people may be highly qualified to help and we're grateful for their role, but do we really want to rely *exclusively* on someone for something—anything—if they've never been through it themselves?

A great percentage of women in the U.S. spend two to four years after high school in education and preparation for the workplace. We are even willing to take out enormous loans for the cause.

Then when it comes to motherhood, we throw ourselves into the most important role of our lives with no study or training—subject to tremendous influence from the medical industry, Hollywood, and other commercial enterprises—reliant on professionals to do it for us, whether "it" is conceiving, birthing, or raising children.

Doesn't our role as mother and homemaker deserve as much commitment, study, and investment as we give to any job in the workplace?

Many people I interviewed had seen or helped with births—even saved moms' and babies' lives. But of those who had, only a handful had seen an all-natural birth in a hospital, much less a home birth, and forget a first home birth with a 42-year-old woman. Of those who could discuss nutrition at length, none of them other than my TCM doctor attended to the role of nutrition to the extent that I did.

What I discovered in my journey of study and in creating my own approach to conception, pregnancy, home birth, and motherhood, I gladly share with you. I don't give medical advice and wouldn't try to tell you what *your* path to a healthy, sacred birth is.

But if you're like I was—with your intuition hinting that

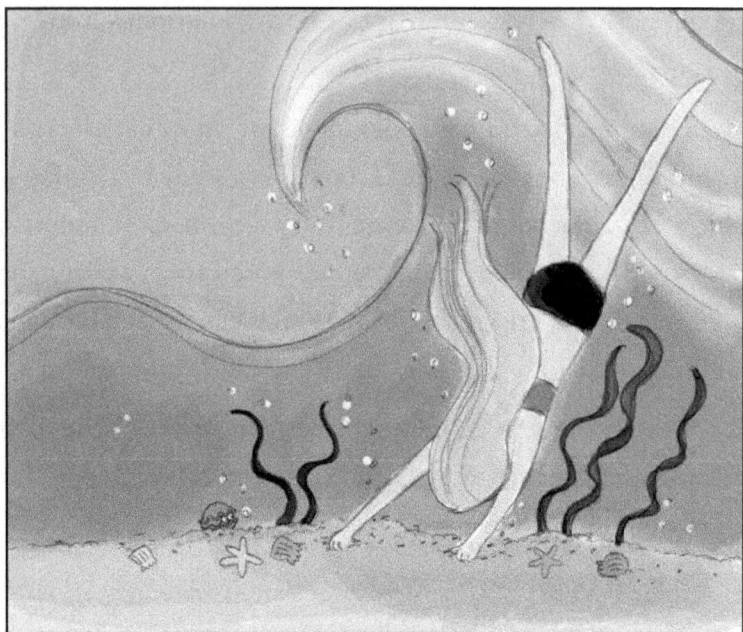

Natural labor is like swimming in the big surf:
dig in and let the waves roll over you.

something better than the norm is possible—but without knowing what a doula really does, not knowing what really qualifies a midwife, and certainly not knowing what kind of help you'll need postpartum (but hopefully knowing you will need some), I've got lots of ideas for you based on *learning* and *doing* myself.

I can do what women have done around the world in all countries since people started talking (and everyone knows we women-folk are good at that). I can tell you my stories, what I learned, and what I came to expect. I hope it will inspire women who want to create their own magical birth experience.

Swimming in the Bliss of Natural Childbirth: My Home Birth Story

Birth is completely natural. My body and my baby know what to do. Together we will do our best to prepare and to build our strength. Then we will let nature do her thing!

Ah, Mother Nature. Just because she knows what to do and will take charge doesn't mean that it won't be incredibly difficult. My throat (among other things) was so sore from grunting and growling in labor that I could barely speak the next day. However, in the big picture that was over in the blink of an eye—yet the reward for my baby and me will last for a lifetime.

If it had just been for me, perhaps painkillers would have been tempting, despite knowing the multiple benefits of natural birth for the mother. But I also wanted my baby to experience her birth and first few days out of the womb with bright eyes and a clear mind.

I'd watched the movie *Orgasmic Birth* a dozen times for fun and inspiration. Though I actually believed that it could happen that way, no, crowning did not feel like an orgasm. But I was prepared ahead of time for the fact that it must be incredibly painful—otherwise how could all my strong friends have chosen drugs and surgery when they were originally so opposed?

There was only one way to make my dream of a blissful, sacred birth happen… and that was to give myself no choice. If I stayed at home, when push came to shove (!), I would have no way to do it but go through it.

Just like swimming in the surf.

All lovers of the ocean know that to reach the open water, you need the courage to leave the shore and swim through the breakwater. This metaphor should not let our minds drift to the warm ankle-slapping waves of the Caribbean. We're talking about Mavericks and Waimea Bay here! When the waves between the shore and the open water are huge, you must dive right into them and let them roll over you. It can be terrifying, but with solid resolve, you reap the reward of an experience few people have.

My original reason for pursuing home birth was only to be able to preserve my goal of a natural, drug-free birth. As I studied more and more, however, I found that a home birth in every way offered the opportunity for a deeply sacred experience. Which it most certainly was.

When I first spoke to my midwife, I asked if she thought I were "high-risk" for home birth. She looked surprised.

"High-risk? Why? Are you sick? Do you have a problem?"

"No," I answered. "But I had two first-trimester miscarriages."

"So?" she replied. "That is a terribly painful experience, but there are millions of miscarriages before babies are born. If it were three or four, we'd have to do further evaluation, but two doesn't necessarily make you high-risk."

"And I have fibroids, though my OB-GYN said they were small and not positioned in a way that would cause a problem."

"OK, that's good. What else?"

"Well, I'm 42 years old."

"Women have always had babies in their 40s. Nothing new there. Are you fit?"

"Yes."

"Do you eat well?"

"Yes."

"Is this what you want?"

"Yes."

"Then of course you can have a home birth."

I asked her to explain the differences in experience and risk between a home birth and a birthing center. The only difference, she assured me, was that (given my home and the birth center were equal distance from an excellent hospital) at the facility, I would not be alone with my husband in my own peaceful environment—and four hours after delivery I would have to pack up, walk to the car with my baby and drive home. At home, four hours after delivery she and her team would have tucked my husband, baby, and me warmly in our bed, fed us, cleaned up, and quietly left.

My husband and I looked at each other, smiled, and both shouted, "Home birth!"

And so it happened. Eight hours after we realized I was in labor, my baby was born in a tub in our family room. The lights were dim, the room warm. My husband had a fire going in our wood-burning oven and traditional Japanese flute music I love wafting through the stereo. He also served as my "squat chair" in the tub.

Surrounded by our midwife and three doulas who stood back until they knew they were needed, my husband and I joked, kissed, and played together right until the intense pushing started. One hour later my baby was born and I was lying on my yoga mat, pushing out the placenta while my baby crawled her way from my abdomen to my breast and started nursing.

Just as they'd said, four hours later we were tucked in bed, the midwives had cleaned the house, and the three of us fell asleep in an ocean of bliss.

That's a summary… not the whole story. It was a blissful birth—everything I wanted and more—but it wasn't easy and it wasn't without moments of great concern. Was there an "emergency"? Without the right midwife—someone who'd delivered hundreds of babies, who'd seen hundreds of "complications" and unexpected events and knew how to respond, someone who'd constantly affirmed my faith and resolve—it might have been.

That is why I was so happy that I'd been patient, that I'd kept looking even at eight months pregnant still determined to find the OB-GYN, midwife, doula, and postpartum doula that would make up my team. Without the team I so carefully selected, the birth would not have gone the way it did.

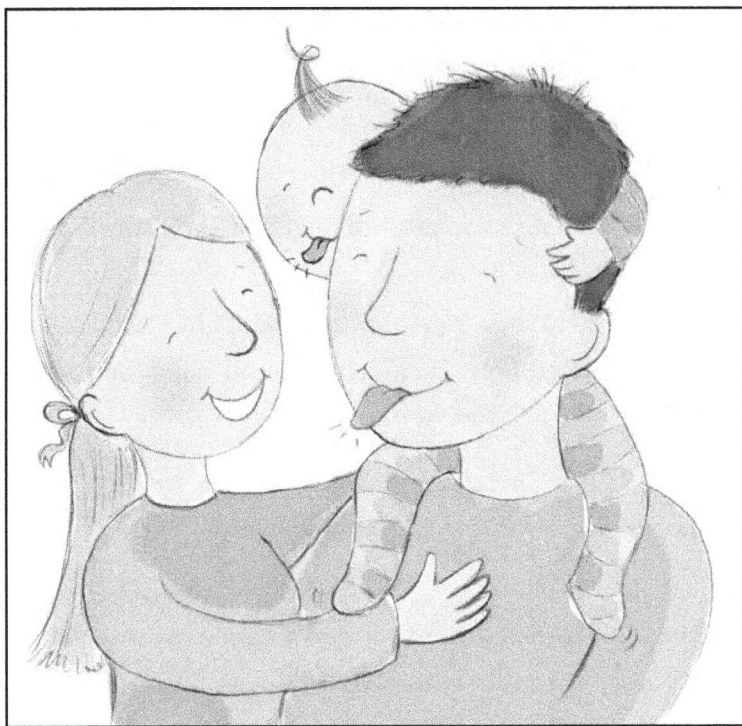

*The postpartum year can be a magical time for the new family...
and having the right help makes that more likely!*

FREEDOM TO CHOOSE

We women folk have never had so much freedom as in the United States today.

We have all the choices we want. Unlike millions of women around the world and throughout history (even recent history in the States), we can do, act, dress, think, eat, date, marry, work, have children (or not) and raise them, all as we choose.

But with all the freedom comes a price.

Without the structure of a cultural system and expectation of the role of women and family, we've been left to figure it out on our own. Further, when it comes to motherhood, there are countless influences (all seeking their own gain, not ours).

These influences are profit driven and determined to tell us how to do it—whether conceiving or delivering our kids, how to feed them, how to school and discipline them, what to buy them, how to dress them, and on and on. Where do we find help navigating the choices and making the most positive healthy decisions?

For many people, the answer is: Nowhere.

Yet it's so common now that it's hardly questioned. It is shocking how women in this country are now left to their own devices in all aspects of parenting. In no country and no time have women been so isolated, uninformed, and left to carry, deliver, and raise their families completely on their own.

In gaining all our freedoms, we lost something major—which some would call a primary need of human beings: Community. With all the joy, love, help, and support it offers.

Gone is the village of women—close family members, neighbors and friends who work together, cook together, swap stories over tea while meals bake—who help one another with the questions and needs that arise daily in raising a family.

Gone is the local midwife who delivered your baby, your sister's babies, your neighbors' babies, and every baby in town.

And gone is the highly skilled domestic help who could support us in a million ways during pregnancy and postpartum.

This partially explains why great numbers of women (almost 50% in some states) have, and even schedule, C-sections (on the encouragement of their doctor), fail to breast feed for long (if at all), rush back on their feet rather than recovering postpartum, resume working as quickly as possible after childbirth,[2] place very young infants in daycare or with nannies, make frozen dinners and fast food meals for their family, leave their infant alone in cribs at night with pharmaceutical formulas and plastic pacifiers in their mouth even in their first month of life, sit their children in front of mind-numbing TV, and overpay unqualified and skill-less domestic help.

No surprise then that we see so many depressed mothers postpartum. This reality would make motherhood depressing. Yet many women don't find support for doing things differently. And there have been at least three generations of women since the circumstances were significantly different.

Do we need to lose our freedom to regain community, to help one another and bring back the joy of motherhood and family?

---

2. Some mothers return to work quickly because they want to—which is their right. Some mothers return to work quickly because they genuinely need the income to survive. And there are people willing to make changes in their physical standard of living so they can reduce their income and outgo to stay at home and care for their children.

There's no turning back time, and I doubt many of us would want to surrender the freedom we have been enjoying. So is there a middle ground? Did we have to throw out all support and community in the name of freedom and progress? I say:

"No! We *can* enjoy our freedoms and find ways to rebuild our village."

"Yes! We *can* support mothers, and retain a healthy, intact family life!"

I was fortunate to have the help I did and that all worked out for the best. But I was on my own researching on the Internet, preparing for the worst, expecting the best, and following my heart with each new challenge along the way. It wasn't easy, and it wasn't achieved without going down a few dead ends and making mistakes.

It is my hope that this book will help women—through all aspects of their pregnancy, delivery, and postpartum—get the best help to realize their dream of motherhood. It is in the spirit of community that I offer what I have learned.

Part 1:

❖ ❖ ❖

Pregnancy

&

Labor and Delivery

Chapter One

Why Do We Need a Doula or a Midwife?

If you are not planning your birth—meaning you are using the template that's been prepared for you by institutions, corporations, and commercially-funded committees—the odds are extremely high that:

• You will notice your contractions are regular, time them, and realize you're *really* in labor.

• You'll call your doctor, her/his secretary or answering service will page her/him, and you'll then receive a call back from either your doctor or another on the team whom you may or likely have not met.

• You'll drive nervously on the freeway to your hospital when you think the contractions are close enough.

- Your contractions may decrease, because the body can slow or reverse its processes under added stress during labor. If they've slowed too much or the cervix has contracted (which can also happen when experiencing stress), you will be sent home and told to wait until the contractions reach certain regularity again. (Many women have repeated this step two times or more.)

An acquaintance of mine, in labor with her first child and with a heart set on natural childbirth in the hospital, was sent home. She and her husband ran out of gas on the freeway making their trip back to the hospital the second time. Her husband fixed his goof, but obviously the stress of rushing back and forth on the freeway, and now running out of gas, had an effect on the mom. Her labor, already delayed from the first trip to the hospital, slowed again. She walked and walked, a full thirty hours to get that baby moving. Finally the hospital intervened with drugs.

- When you return to the hospital, you will either be placed in a wheelchair or you will walk to a labor room. The routine is being hooked up to an IV, one or several monitors, denied food and even beverages (other than ice chips, which in many cultures are considered something to avoid in labor).

Depending on how "progressive" the hospital and staff are, you will be allowed or encouraged to walk around and work different labor positions to encourage the baby into the correct position and allow labor to progress, or you will simply be advised to stay flat on your back—which is considered by midwives (and many mothers) to be one of the most painful and least effective ways to labor.

• Around the time you start experiencing stronger contractions and the pain sensations are increasing, hospital staff (more strangers) armed with drugs and needles will begin to appear at your door offering "relief." I've heard of them saying, "It doesn't need to feel like this. We can make that pain go away." Surely not for everyone, but for me that would be the equivalent of a thief coming to steal a sacred moment and opportunity for growth.

At this point in labor, an acquaintance of mine who delivered in a hospital in Sacramento asked her nurse for an extra pillow and the nurse responded, "Only one pillow per room." This same hospital played, "Rock-a-Bye Baby" (yes, the classic bizarre song in which the baby and cradle fall to the ground) every time a woman in the ward delivered, and streamed the music into every labor room for other laboring mothers to hear.

• You will be checked periodically by doctors, residents, and/or nurses and student nurses. When you're dilated far enough, they will move you to the delivery room where your doctor, or a stand-in if he or she has been called away to more pressing matters, will stay with you as the baby and the placenta are born.

This is all assuming that you're not put on additional drugs to speed labor (if in their estimation you're taking too long). While 24 hours is a common length of time for a mother—especially with her first baby—to labor, many hospitals encourage drugs to speed the process if it passes 12 hours.

It is also assuming that nothing has happened to encourage the doctor to perform a cesarean section (now at 30-50% of deliveries in the States, varying by doctor and hospital).

• After the baby and placenta are born, they are both taken away in most instances. The baby to be washed (unnecessary and considered by many to be stressful for the newborn who'd rather be on her mother's chest), weighed, measured, and treated with various pharmaceutical products.

The placenta will be taken to an incinerator.

Observing a birth in a hospital in Dallas, I watched as the placenta (considered by some a sacred organ that supported the baby's life for nine months and a healing medicine for the mother to consume) was dropped on the floor (with a highly uncomfortable splat) in front of the mother and baby. The nurse said, "Whoops" and bent down to scoop it into a metal bowl.

And finally, over the next day or two, the mother will be offered formula samples, fed with processed and microwaved foods, questioned and (along with her baby) prodded by more strangers (hospital staff and students). Then they'll be sent home. And that's it.

Whoa!

How has the most sacred rite of passage become so cold and offensive?

Where's the romance, the beauty, the nurturing?

There are countless studies documenting the value of a natural, peaceful childbirth for the mother and baby—but let's just consider common sense:

You—an adult, calloused and accustomed to the harshness life can serve up, arrive for your first day in a new house. On the way there your real estate agent offers you a beverage so you can relax—but something's been slipped into the drink so you're not seeing clearly and you're feeling disoriented. On entering you're doused with chilled water and placed under floodlights in a cold room while strangers probe, prod, prick, and monitor you. Then you're sequestered in a corner of the house in a big plastic bed where you "rest" for a few days to sleep off the hangover before you can really enjoy your new home and be with your family.

Where's the love?

At most hospitals, it's been erased by procedures created by administrators, accountants, lawyers, and insurance companies—moneymakers all.

Are there hospitals and staff working in them who sincerely care for the mother and her experience? There are some, and I found such a doctor and a hospital (after months of looking and interviews) in the event my midwife decided we needed to transfer.

But how much time do pregnant parents usually have to invest in determining if the hospital they choose supports women's choices and desires for a natural, peaceful birth experience? And once they find that doctor or nurse who understands their desires, the parents can't even count on them to be available when the mother goes into labor.

We can all see the need for a different approach and the need for support—for someone who understands the needs of, and advocates for, the mother. A person with whom she's met, established rapport and trust, and whom she knows will be there when the big moment arrives. Someone who's not a friend, mother-in-law, nor the father—they have different roles.

We need a person who has witnessed and participated in hundreds of births to represent our best interest and desires in the heat of the moment. Many hospital staff members will make it seem as if there are no alternatives to things such as laboring on your back, fetal monitors, IVs, forceps, wearing the hospital "gown" and ice-chip-only rules.

We need someone who understands hospital procedures and possible alternatives.

That person is a midwife or a doula.

And whether you're like me and think that home is the safest, happiest place to have your baby, or you believe you'll feel better cared for and safer in a hospital—either way, you'll want a midwife and/or doula.

Chapter Two

The Role of a Doula and How to Find One

The Role of a Doula

There are many differences between a midwife and a doula. If you're going to have a home birth, you'll have at least one of each and they're both vitally important in different ways. Your midwife will be in charge of the delivery, and she may arrive early in your labor or not. Your doula, however, should come to your house as soon as you know you're in labor; she will stay with you the entire time, and usually four hours or more after the birth. She is also the person who will visit you one or several times during the next few days.

So while your midwife is experienced in delivering babies and will be the leader on your big day, you'll actually spend more time with your doula.

If you're going to have a hospital birth, you can have a midwife or doula working for you, but even if she is a midwife, she'll have to serve as a "doula only" in the hospital—because only the OB-GYN can actually "catch" the baby (they say they "deliver" the baby—ha!).

A doula, generally speaking, is a birth coach—coach meaning someone experienced in what you're wanting to achieve who assists you physically and emotionally to achieve it.

I also like to call them "translators." You might say in labor, "ahhhhel–nooooo." She knows that means to tell the visiting person offering drugs to kindly leave the room. Or you reply with a grunt to your husband's helpful advice. Your doula's translation: "I think she'd love it if you rub her back—quietly."

Anyone can serve as your doula—from a ready-to-faint father to a woman who is certified and has apprenticed under a midwife for years or decades.[3] Later we'll discuss in detail why the latter is the better choice.

Doula comes from the Greek, meaning "a woman who serves." What is a servant, or "one who serves?" In the U.S. we have no idea. To begin with, it's no longer considered polite or appropriate to use the word "servant," and of those who work in a servant capacity, only a few deserve the title.

---

3. The doula training programs in the U.S. (such as offered by DONA— Doulas of North America) cover important material and help maintain the integrity of the profession—but we still want a doula with lots and lots of experience.

I call out the U.S. as a place where service is no longer appreciated or commonly provided based on my experience around the world. It's true in all areas of service: the hospitality industry, domestic help, childcare, elder care, personal/body care, etc. If you are unfamiliar with excellent service, go on this little adventure:

> Fly an American airline and ask the attendant for extravagant and decadent service—to bring you an extra plastic cup of tap water. Sit in the American airline's terminal, lounge, use the bathroom, and ask for a change in seat assignment.
>
> Next, do the same thing on Singapore Airlines, Cathay Pacific, or even Hava Yollari (Turkish Airlines). You'll see what I mean. You will feel like Saul—knocked over, scales falling from your eyes, now seeing the light.

A servant is a person who serves, who provides a service. That means that if we work at jobs either in the home or outside the home, we are servants. If we provide that service with love and honor, then we are excellent servants and deserve to be rewarded richly with the pleasure of honorable work, financial abundance, and choices (in case we're not being rewarded appropriately).

Servant is a title that deserves the utmost respect, if the title has been earned with sufficient training, dedication, and delivered with excellence.

Something else that was thrown out with the use of the word *servant* was the actual role. Full-time servants, reserved now for only the very wealthiest, are no longer a part of the family scene, having been replaced with maids—women doing only a decent or tolerable job who come once every week or two, and babysitters (often less qualified than even the maids), many of whom plant themselves, the children, and donuts in front of the TV the moment the parents leave.[4]

The New York Times best-selling book and blockbuster movie *The Help* shows much more than how unfairly and often cruelly the servants were treated in the South in the '60s. It also shows how *infinitely* more competent the servants were at cooking, cleaning, and caring for children than those ladies-of-the-house and mothers, and more competent than today's servants.

And why were they so much better? They had learned skills watching and listening to their mothers who had learned (to varying degrees how to cook, bake, present beautiful meals, launder, iron and mend fine fabrics, polish silver, grocery shop, and care for children—even potty and sleep training) from their mothers and had years of practice.

---

4. Further examples of such talent: During the process of finding my excellent nanny, one woman applied for the position boasting of her experience dog-sitting; another of her 9 years cheerleading (photo posing seductively in uniform included as evidence); and a third of having a little brother.

The irony is that they were paid a pittance for those incredible gifts they brought to the family, while today's candidates, often freshly unemployed from every other form of work—people without skills, however well-educated—are grossly overpaid. (I'm generalizing, but with good reason; bear with me. There are also loving and highly intelligent, worthy, and noble servants, but it takes a while to find them—and even then they usually need much more training).

Without extended families, and with so-so maids and babysitters, everyone loses (except the so-so's). The problem is not that people are incapable. It's the lack of training, the low expectations, and lack of respect for the roles by those who fill them as well as those who employ them.

If the role of a highly-trained, multi-talented servant were expected and respected, it would encourage women (and men in varying roles) to learn again the craft and art of service and teach it to their children.

Who am I to be saying all this? For starters, I grew up in the South in the '60s and '70s (and while Texas doesn't consider itself the South, Texans sure carry the attitudes of southerners).

Like those servants in the Old South, I learned to cook and clean from my mama, a hard-working single mom, who even when I was eight and a bit too short, showed me how, with a stool, to reach the sink and cook, clean, and do laundry. She taught me how and required that I practice.

The cooking skills that she passed on she'd learned from her family. They left a lot to be desired and made the Campbell's soup company a bit richer. However, that petite woman could scrub something scary, could make a bed with sheet corners so perfect they could cut, and no drawer, closet, or bed had as much as a stray sock stuffed under or thrown in it. The house—inside and out, up and down—sparkled.

Perhaps most importantly, muttering, grumbling, or complaining while cleaning was cause for a lecture and loss of privileges (like a ride to school). Her mantra was, "DAMN-IT-TO-HELL, I SAID *WHISTLE* WHILE YOU WORK!"

Naturally, as a child I was ungrateful for this great training, but it's easy to see—by anyone with a sense of accomplishment and drive—that it was invaluable.

I cleaned houses for a living while in school and even after college. After working for a few years in the financial markets earning up to $20,000 per month (a noteworthy income back in the early '90s—and even now), I decided to take a break and actually *enjoy* what I did for work again—so I started another cleaning business.

I think this story is illustrative:

I had been lying on the beach every day for a few months when I decided it was time to start doing something creative again. I looked in the newspaper (1996, when a few people still read them) and saw a cleaning business for sale.

The gentleman who answered my call explained that he "really didn't have a business to sell."

"Well, you ran an ad. What for?"

"I have a vacuum cleaner and the phone number of a lady I cleaned house for."

"A used vacuum and a phone number? You ran a newspaper ad to sell that!"

"It's not much. But the lady I cleaned for is rich and has a lot of rich friends. If she likes what you do, you'll get a lot of business."

"I'll give you $50 for the vacuum and the number." So it was settled.

I called the rich woman, arranged a meeting, and showed up with a new vacuum (since I'd been able to start my new business so cheaply, I went out on a limb and bought a new $800 Miele, not wanting to disgrace myself or offend someone intelligent by entering their home with the dusty piece I received from the initial investment).

During the first meeting we established her needs and that I could more than satisfy them. My business had begun.

Within six months, just as the man with the vacuum predicted, I had received multiple referrals from that one client, and then multiple referrals from all of them. Within six months I had over fifty residential and commercial accounts, all without any advertising. Soon I had trained excellent women to work with me, and I was right back on that beach every afternoon.

I did have a college degree and diverse business experience, but those skills are irrelevant in the role of maid, and in no manner merit higher pay than someone who, perhaps, has no schooling and has never done anything but clean. A diploma is great and I'm happy to have mine—but as proof of qualification and ability? I wouldn't wipe my counter with that paper. Skills, drive, and talent, please!

What impressed my clients is that, as my mama taught me—by golly—I could clean a house. There was nothing that escaped me. There were things I cleaned that clients would never have thought of, noticed, or known to do themselves. And when I told them they needed an all-day spring-cleaning (at any time of year) with three maids for $400, they didn't bat an eye. They knew they were going to get $800 worth of clean.

Although I'd always ask what they wanted, my clients did not need to ask or direct me. I knew what to do, I went the extra mile, and they would find their homes sparkling, fresh, and inviting.

My trademark was the bowl of fresh citrus—which would have been simply irritating if done in a house that was cleaned marginally. But in a house that was spotless, imagine a bowl of fresh citrus, picked from my trees (stem and leaves attached), washed and placed in the center of the client's dining table in one of their most beautiful bowls under a crystal chandelier showering yellows, oranges, and greens with delicate light.

Yep, my clients loved me and I loved them. The work I did was an expression of love and respect. I did it well and I whistled while I worked.

And now understanding a little more about service and servants, back to our doulas...

Ancient Chinese medical texts advise that a woman must spend her pregnancy in a peaceful environment, enjoying only things of beauty and absorbing (through her company, environment, and reading sacred books) peaceful thoughts and higher knowledge.

Here are just a few examples:

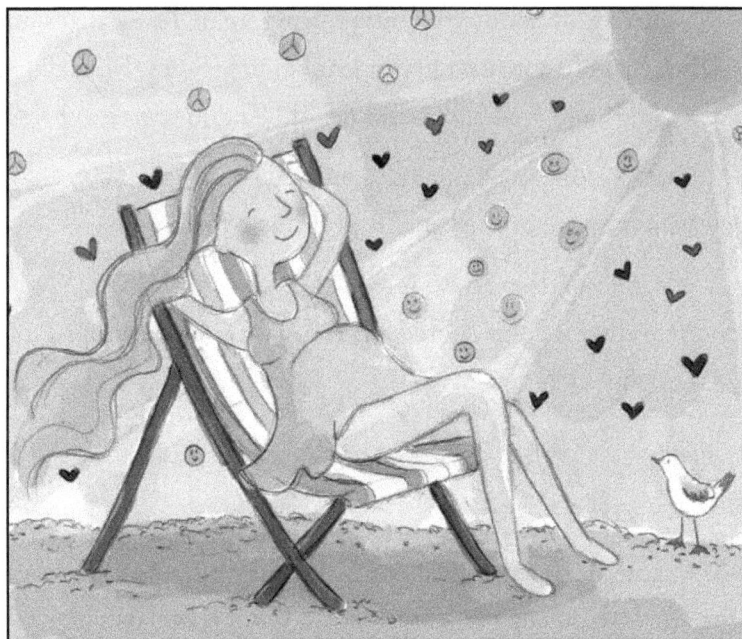

*The ancients advised that pregnant women should spend time in a beautiful and peaceful environment, **tended by handsome servants**, no less.*

A pregnant woman carries with her the finest piece of jade [the baby]. She should enjoy all things, look at fine pictures, and be attended by handsome servants.

From Admonitions to Ladies

She should eat no odd-tasting food, see no ugly scenes, and listen to no licentious sounds.

From Ladies of Virtue

I don't know about you, but growing up in Texas, that's not exactly how the average woman spent her pregnancy. Most didn't have servants and we'd sure never heard of a dou-*what?*

That's slowly changing, and women are becoming increasingly aware of the benefits of hiring a birth doula.

The role of the doula is whatever the mother and doula decide together the role should be. Today the job of a professional doula usually includes:

1.) Understanding deeply the physical and emotional needs of a woman in labor.

A father is not the ideal doula. He may offer great support, help, and love during the labor process, but it is *his* labor process, too. Because he is deeply involved emotionally, and because he doesn't have experience supporting a mother in labor (and one or two previous births don't come close to making either parent truly experienced), he should be free to simply support the mother (and himself) with loving physical contact and encouragement—not with labor coaching or shuttling as an intermediary with hospital staff.

For similar reasons, friends and other family members are not the ideal doulas.

A doula *works* for the mother. She's hired and paid to support, to be an intermediary (not to replace) medical staff, and to do exactly as the mother wishes. Ideally having extensive experience, a doula can understand and even anticipate the physical and emotional feelings and needs a mother goes through in labor and has a "tool kit" of ways to best respond to those needs. Knowing that, the mother is more likely to listen calmly to the doula when the need arises.

A doula acts as an orchestra conductor for the family, allowing the father, friends, and other family members to be present for the concert—and involved to the degree that they and the mother want them to be. This takes stress off everyone's shoulders, removing their uncertainty about "doing it the right way," thus enabling everyone to participate joyfully.

2.) Helping the mother understand the process and to design a birth plan.

If a mother is planning a hospital birth and intends to give birth naturally with the least intervention possible, she will need to know what procedures are going to be encouraged (if not forced on her), and which ones she will be able to decline or modify.

An experienced doula will be aware of the procedures and practices of local hospitals and will be able to help the mother plan.

A birth plan is a written document that *should be read* and respected by your doctor and/or hospital staff, but according to my doulas that isn't always the case (if the plan is too long, poorly written, etc.). Your doula can help you write a brief and concise plan that is more likely to be read, respected, and followed.

3.) Helping the mother achieve her birth plan by coaching her and acting as an intermediary between her and her family or, in the case of a hospital birth, between her and the staff.

For a home birth, the doula almost always works in complete harmony with the midwife, and both work to best achieve the woman's birth plan.

In the OB-GYN and hospital world, birth plans are often discouraged, frowned upon, or simply ignored. When I told the first OB-GYN I interviewed that I had heard doulas were very helpful and asked if she could recommend one to help me with my birth plan and to coach me during labor, she said, "Sure, I'll email contact information to you." The email never came. When I called her office to follow-up and ask about it, no return phone call. I switched doctors.

(Note: your doctor, as I learned, is not the person to ask for a referral for a midwife or doula—more on that later.)

Whether they are sincerely working in what they believe are the mother's best interests or not, doctors are generally not enthusiastic about being told how to do their job—which is how they view a birth plan. There are always exceptions, but mothers must often dedicate a great amount of time interviewing to find doctors who support truly natural birth experiences in the hospital environment.

The third OB-GYN I found, at seven months pregnant, was by far the most understanding, respectful, and nurturing. He offered me a chair in his office for an hour-long conversation in

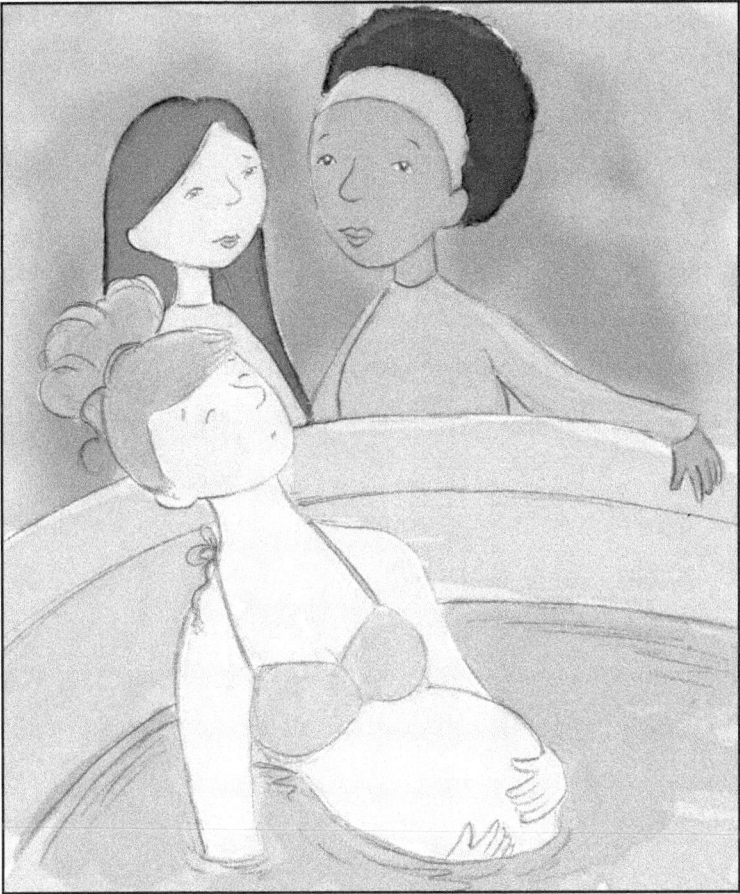

In a home birth, the doula and midwife work in harmony to help achieve the mother's goals.

our first meeting. (The other two had their assistants get me naked and in stirrups before introducing themselves and conducting a ten minute inspection of my genital area.)

He listened to my list of wishes regarding a natural birth and seemed to genuinely support them. However, when I asked him about bringing my doula or midwife to the hospital with me and having them help write my birth plan, he said, "Oh, you won't need that."

Often one will hear that with a natural childbirth in a hospital, the mother gets the best of both (natural and the medical scenarios); that even deeply-entrenched doctors and nurses can be persuaded, eventually, to listen to and adhere to the mother's wishes, once the mother has shown strong determination and is clear about what she wants.

Say huh?

Some laboring moms may be interested in courtroom antics to engender respect from the hospital staff. But if you want to be in a hospital without needing to prove you know what you want and need for your birth experience, a doula can serve you well.

If you would like to labor squatting, walking, or in the shower...

If you would like an intimate and private environment (no strangers walking into your room periodically to encourage drug use or residents "checking" you—your vitals and cervix, to be exact)...

If you want to play special music...

If you want to be offered your own beverages and foods during labor...

If you want to wear your own clothes rather than a rough and ugly, half-open hospital gown...

If you want to be free to laugh, scream, or cry as loudly as you need...

If you want someone you know and trust at your side at all times to massage, assist, or simply hold your hand...

It is the job of your doula to help make sure your desires are met.

(In the case of monitors, IVs, food, beverage, music, and labor positions—rules vary from hospital to hospital about what is forced, what is allowed, and what can be declined. Your doula should know your hospital's policies and the two of you should prepare for them ahead of time.)

If there is a nurse or any staff member whom you'd rather not see in your room again for *whatever reason*, your doula will see to that. If you need another blanket or pillow—you don't need to beg a nurse and be told you've already reached your pillow quota—your doula will find one.

When you think you're surely dying and perhaps do need

drugs, your doula is there to comfort and encourage you. To tell you that you're doing great, that even if you claim you're close to death with each contraction, it's normal, perfect, and all is going according to what you dreamed!

Note: It's a good idea to discuss with your doula ahead of time how she should respond if you change your plan when the pain peaks. I told my midwife, "I can take it. If I'm acting like I want to veer from my plan, that will only be fear talking. You can soothe or yell at me, or both—whatever it takes to keep me on course."

Other mothers may tell a doula, *if I change my mind and want drugs, help me get them ASAP*, and that's what the doula should do.

More than once I looked up at my doula and asked with all the fear and hope in the world, "Can I really do this?" She'd look at me with the calmest, most confident eyes and say, "Yes. You *are* doing it." And that was all I needed to get to the next phase.

At the peak of labor—that golden moment called crowning—my doula told me I needed to push at least three times per contraction. (Apparently I was only pushing twice.)

It was the only time I hung my head and cried, "But I can't push anymore!"

She said with a smile, "You can't stop now. That baby's head is out!"

She didn't need to tell me twice.

You're getting the idea here. You don't want to go into labor without your doula!

HOW TO FIND A DOULA

Even if you are deeply entrenched in your community and have numerous friends who have chosen home or natural birth in a hospital and have a doula to recommend, you still may need to look to the electronic village to find the doula who's a perfect match for you.

But before you jump online, sit down and visualize the perfect birth. What do you want? The answers will vary with every woman. For consideration, here was my list:

The Environment:

I want to have my baby at home, with a fire going, beautiful music playing, and my husband by my side.

The Help:

Midwife: I want an incredibly experienced midwife. For me, that means she would have attended hundreds of births and delivered not dozens, but *hundreds* of babies.

To trust my health and the health of my baby in the hands of anyone less experienced would be unthinkable. She must have an established practice, numerous references, and partners with whom she works whom I trust to the exact degree that I trust and click with her (in the event two births happen at the same time and the midwife is occupied with the other birth—very rare with midwives who schedule properly).

She must not only be highly experienced and talented, she must be patient, kind, nurturing, clearly understand and agree with my directives and desires, and we must "click" instantly.

The Doula:

I want a doula who is equally experienced in her role. No rookies getting paid training on my clock! She must be highly disciplined, responsive, punctual, accountable, and fun. She must love what she does, but must consider it work and approach it as a business.

Here's why:

In any job where there is no bar to entry and a good living to be made, you will find a whole spectrum of people: those working well, the so-so's, and those pretending to work. Consider these professions: flight attendant, cook, preacher, yoga teacher, massage therapist, real estate agent, writer, and many more.

Some of these professions, like doula and midwife, will have one or more organizations that certify or even license practitioners, which is important. But does that mean these people are *good* at their job?

Take even a medical doctor...

I had a friend whose cousin, though she did decently in medical school, had just failed her medical boards for the fifth time. Did I accidentally type fifth when I meant to type first? 5th!

She called my friend to say, "I've just been partying too much to keep focused. I know I can pass. Can I come stay at your house for a few months and study before I try again?"

And what happened when she got to his house? She just started partying in a different city and continued studying with hangovers.

Naturally she failed again. But apparently that's no problem—she can just keep-on takin' that exam until she manages to pass. To be fair, some folks just aren't real good at taking exams, but would you line up for appointments with them?

While we do want to work with people who have displayed at least the minimum effort and talent in their chosen position by getting the certificates, licenses, and/or other government issued papers, what matters far, far more than that is *years* of experience. In-the-field training. The old-timey word for that is *apprenticeship*.

In ancient China, and even as recently as the last 50 years, it was unacceptable for a person to call themselves a "Traditional Chinese Medicine Doctor" unless they'd apprenticed for years and years under a respected, usually elderly (and thus, richly experienced) doctor. Often, TCM doctors come from lines of doctors going back in their families for three to thirty generations.

That approach, true apprenticeship, doesn't fly in America anymore. Is it that apprenticeship fails to offer an ideal path to learning? No, it's because nobody wants to devote the time (traditionally, for a few to several years) to *really* learn and gain that crucial experience. They want to start raking in the dough immediately.

I wouldn't want a doctor or health provider who's been practicing less than 30 years—and preferably a third generation doctor in a family where practice had been a topic of conversation from childhood.

In Germany they have a similar approach to mine—even to baking bread! One must attend a special school to study baking before assuming the title of baker or opening a bakery. We don't need to follow the German example in many instances, but one has to admire a people who so respect their bread that they require special training to earn the title Baker. (And the bread there is, without fail, extraordinary.)

Back in the U.S., anyone, and I mean *anyone* who says, I am a doula, midwife, postpartum doula, maid, cook, or nanny… is. But do we want them working for us?

The average doula will earn between $500–$1,000 for a

few meetings and one day's work. That's decent pay for someone highly qualified, but serious cash for someone mediocre who left a kindergarten teacher job and decided to go for the big money as a doula.

After writing an outline of your perfect birth scenario, the next step is to call referrals you've received from friends, or go online to search for doulas.

The first thing when speaking with them—before even meeting them—is to ask them to write a single paragraph about what makes them unique and email it to you.

You'd be shocked at how many people will not even go to that trouble. This is a good first step in determining who prides themselves in their work, can take direction well, who is literate, professional, and willing to invest a few minutes to earn your business. With those who send an email (and you like what they wrote), go to the next step of scheduling a meeting and have your list of questions. I would have already determined on the first phone call that they had years of experience and assisted in at least fifty births.

I would ask:

- What do you consider most important in your role as birth doula?

- How do you handle a mother changing her birth plan in the middle of the birth?

- How do you handle a doctor or hospital staff member trying to encourage a laboring mother to do something against her birth plan?

- Tell me the story of a birth you attended that went perfectly.

- Tell me the story of a birth that had complications and changes in plan, and tell me how you responded.

- How long after I call and leave a message for you can I expect to hear back?

- How do you schedule your clients so you can guarantee you'll be available to attend my birth?

- Are you planning to travel during my due date period, or can you guarantee you'll be in town and available?

- Who is your backup in case you're not available? When can I have a meeting with her/them? (I would insist on meeting the back-up and knowing I feel comfortable with her/them as well. I would not share my sacred day with someone I'd never seen.)

- What is included in your fee? How many prenatal and postpartum visits and what is involved?

- What is your refund policy if we change direction or if you and/or your partner are not available when I go into labor?

This is just an outline. Design your own list of questions based on your needs.

If you do not have the funds to pay for a doula, there are sometimes programs at hospitals in which doulas-in-training will serve during labor at no cost.

If you do have the funds, it is preferable to work with an experienced doula... and one who is working for you, not the hospital.

If it is very important for you to work with an experienced doula, that should be the first thing you determine on the phone before taking the time for a meeting. I've been surprised to find websites advising doulas not to be overly concerned in the beginning if they don't have much experience yet because "so many people don't even ask."

I'm sure most doulas would not try to hide their lack of experience, but I also believe that many would try to go it on their own before having apprenticed for very long. Remember, *they* might think they're a pro after attending 20 births and being certified. But I disagree.

I would ask for the exact number of labors they'd attended and participated in, how many they were the primary doula for (different from apprenticing), and for five references. I might not call more than three, but if they can't provide phone numbers for five happy people for whom they've worked, they certainly haven't done a good job or just haven't attended many births.

After you've determined that you're comfortable with the doula's approach and experience, and that you can afford her service, the most important thing is to feel the "click." Is this someone with whom you want to share one of the most magical and intense days of your life?

In my case, I chose my midwife, Selena, first, and then had my choice of the three doulas who worked with her.

The first one was named Pearl. When she was measuring my abdomen and feeling around for my baby, it was like a cat walking on my belly—which felt amazing!

In the car after meeting her the first time, I said to my husband, "I think Daisy was great!"

He asked, "Who's Daisy? Do you mean Pearl?"

I replied, "Who's Pearl?"

From that day on, we called Pearl Daisy, and she accepted her new name amicably.

The next doula I met was Laura. She had curly black and silver hair in two braids that flowed over her shoulders and down her chest. She was the "placenta specialist"—preparing placentas for moms who consider it a rejuvenating supplement to take postpartum (recommended highly in Chinese Medicine and many other cultures). She had a photo album of all the placentas she'd prepared. She lovingly handled each one like a delicate flower. It was amazing how much respect and magic she brought to her job.

I said to my husband, "Laura's an Earth mother! I like her, too. Who better to process the placenta for us!"

My husband was perhaps too queasy to speak, but he smiled and nodded yes.

I met the third doula, Gianna, who looked like an African goddess with dozens of beautiful black and golden braids. She was as warm and beautiful as she looked.

I said to my husband, "I like Gianna, too. Whom do we pick?"

He couldn't decide either.

During one of the appointments with our midwife, she asked if we'd made our decision among Daisy, Laura, and Gianna.

I said, "We can't. We love all three of them."

Selena smiled in her deeply maternal and heartwarming way. "Then if there aren't any other births on your big day, we'll all be there with you."

This exchange about the doulas confirmed what we'd known: that we'd found a loving person who, yes, was being paid for a job, but was doing it because it was her great desire and talent.

Your time with your doula will end very shortly after your

baby is born—maybe in the first day postpartum but almost always in the first week.

That's when your postpartum doula comes into the picture. But wait! If we're having a homebirth, or if we just want someone in the hospital with us who has the extra experience and training, we need to find a midwife.

Chapter Three

The Role of a Midwife and How to Find One

The Role of a Midwife

The midwife helps the mother deliver her baby—at home or in a birthing center. Some midwives are employed by hospitals, but our focus is on those who work delivering in homes or birth centers.

It's my belief that no servant can serve two employers. If a midwife is working for a hospital, that's the employer she's serving. A hospital midwife might be excellent, but for me the purpose of having a midwife is to have someone working in my best interest—and *only* mine.

If a midwife goes with the mother to the hospital, even with her midwife talent and credentials, hospital rules dictate that she can work only in the capacity of doula. But at home, she runs the show—with the mother, of course! That said, midwives sometimes need to transfer the mother to a hospital during labor. They often know all the staff and the rules, so they are excellent "translators" and defenders of the mother's needs.

Historically, every big family or small town had a midwife whom all the women counted on to help deliver their babies. She may have been a trained nurse, someone who worked only as a midwife, or a family member with experience. This was true even in the U.S. until the turn of the 20th century.

That changed because of either manipulation and fear mongering by the medical industry or by exciting medical advancement—depending on one's position—so that now 99% of U.S. births are in hospitals, and approximately 99% of those involve some kind of drug or intervention.

If you have decided to avoid the hospital unless there is a medical emergency or illness, you'll want to find a midwife—and the process is exactly the same as finding a doula.

Midwives may be state licensed as a "certified nurse-midwife," while others who have attended midwifery school are called direct or lay midwives. There is no national academic entry requirement for midwifery courses. Some are covered by insurance and some aren't. Some have years and decades of experience, and some are new to their work.

Many midwives are trained in procedures such as providing oxygen to the mother or newborn, suturing, neonatal resuscitation, and administering oxytocin or other medications for postpartum hemorrhaging (but not for inducing labor).

HOW TO FIND A MIDWIFE

There are websites and agencies that refer midwives in a specific area, but don't assume a midwife is qualified for your needs just because she belongs to certain organizations.

Ask for referrals from agencies and then search online, make phone calls, ask for referrals, and conduct interviews. When you find someone with all the credentials and experience you want and you feel that "click," you've found your midwife.

The first midwife I found to interview came to my home where we spoke for about an hour.

She was very active in the midwife community, promoted her approach to midwifery and encouraged others to follow her protocol. She had two other midwives with whom she worked and who would be backup for me if she were unavailable when I went into labor.

I was four months pregnant when I found her and was really looking forward to establishing a relationship with someone. Perhaps I was too hasty. I didn't have a bad feeling, but I didn't have a great one either. Still, I thought it was good to get that checked off the list. I signed her paperwork and gave her a $700.00 deposit (of a $3,500 total fee). Now I had a midwife and could get to the other hundred things I needed to arrange.

Only a few weeks later my OB-GYN advised that I take a blood glucose test for gestational diabetes. That story could be of great interest to every reader, so I include it at the end of this chapter.

After I'd taken the first test, I was determined to not take the next 100g glucose test. I turned to my midwife for ideas about an alternative approach to the matter.

I told her that I wanted as little testing and intervention as possible, and that under no circumstances did I want to take a test that might determine if something might be "wrong" with the baby that would lead to a "choice" about whether I wanted to "keep" it or not.

She apparently wasn't listening, because in that same meeting she mentioned a recommended medical test during the last weeks of pregnancy that was "optional for women over 40." It checks the baby's responses to the mother's eating and helps determine if the baby could "continue to live" in the womb (or something morbid like that) or if labor should be induced.

Though some women would appreciate it, I had made my desires clear. I was horrified that she would even mention such a thing. It was to avoid a medical and intervention agenda that I was choosing a home birth!

I asked her if there were an alternative. She said, "If you feel the baby kick or move around shortly after you eat, that's the sign they're looking for."

Pregnancy can make you more candid—if you're not careful.

I *wanted* to say, "Perhaps you are one of those people who could be nine months pregnant and not realize you were carrying a child and be wondering what happened to your period—but I'm a little more connected and sensitive than that! I feel it when my baby blinks." I refrained, on the assumption that she was just trying to cover all the bases. After all, there's no reason to be unkind, even when someone's being an idiot.

I should have known right then that it was time to make a change, but it took one more event to make it clear.

On a Thursday morning I called to ask her thoughts about the second gestational diabetes test. She didn't answer her phone, so I left a voicemail. She'd been out of town, so I didn't hear back from her until Monday morning.

I asked, "Don't you leave word on your voicemail that you'll be unavailable for some time and leave a number to contact your alternate (or backup) midwife?"

She said, "I didn't think your message was urgent, so I didn't see that I needed to return the call until Monday when I got back."

Wrong answer! When a pregnant woman calls with a concern about her health and her baby, it may not be an emergency, but it *is* urgent. *Someone* should return the call—ASAP.

She said she hadn't considered changing her outgoing voicemail to let people know when she'd be unavailable, but would think about that in the future.

Wrong answer! If you work in an HR department, you can let people wonder if you even got their voicemail for days and days. In almost any other profession, and certainly for a midwife, if you're unavailable, you leave a way for your clients to reach you or your backup.

I asked why she didn't have her backup call me while she was away. She informed me that since we'd first met three weeks earlier, she'd stopped working altogether with those two women and didn't have a replacement partner yet—but she was working on it.

Very wrong answer! That people change partners in their business is acceptable, but given her other answers, I understood why she wasn't working with the other women anymore... because they didn't want to work with her!

If your midwife (or doula, or health care provider) changes their backup partners, they should notify you immediately and give you the opportunity to meet the new person. Not bothering to do so is a sign of disrespect.

This is another example of how far off the deep end the medical industry has gone—and how complacent or resigned women are to accepting it. Doctors fully expect that they can have any other doctor, whether or not you know or like them, stand in for them, for *the most intimate and important of services.*

I couldn't work with someone who treated me like a car that could be towed into the shop, thrown on a rack, and prodded by any ol' mechanic!

I ask again: *How has the most sacred rite of passage become so cold and offensive?*

When we finally got to the question of the glucose test, my midwife said that there were no alternatives and I would have to take the 100g test.

That was it. I knew I'd rather go it alone than continue working with that midwife. I told her that I felt the way she'd interacted was unprofessional, uncaring, and that my husband and I were going to look for another midwife.

Did she show concern, apologize, and offer a refund? None of the above, and when we asked for a refund of the $700 deposit, she said she'd "turned down other possible clients already" during my birth timeframe, so she couldn't offer even a partial refund.

Every reader will have their own thoughts on how that midwife should have responded, but for me, anyone working in any service capacity should honor their work and their clients. If they've let them down, there should be an apology and some restitution offered (unless the client is outrageous or abusive, but that's a different situation).

I was really fortunate that that exchange occurred so early in my work with her, because it gave me time to start my hunt for a midwife again well before I went into labor!

I searched online and found several other individual and groups of midwives, but nothing was clicking. One was too far away. Another was dear friends with Ina May Gaskin (the goddess of midwifery—read her books!) and revered in the Bay Area, but was retiring from delivering and just lecturing. A third just didn't feel right.

When I saw Selena's website and her photo, I knew she was the one. I could see she was a lioness—strong, in control, but caring and protective. I'm often the tiger in my group, but I knew I'd feel like a cub in her care, which is what I wanted.

Gianna answered my call. She invited us to their monthly open house for people considering home birth or birth at their center.

When my husband and I approached the building on a cold, windy night, we had to cross a very busy street from the parking area. I was a little discouraged imagining this scene when I was in labor, but remembering the photo, I stayed open. Besides, we were here to find out about birth center births and *home births*, which would eliminate the need to deal with traffic, cold or wind, period!

The moment we crossed the threshold, the warm, sure feeling returned and we knew this was the right path.

All the couples in attendance talked about why they were considering home birth, wanting a midwife, and hoping to avoid the hospital. We all had the exact hopes and concerns: a safe, warm, nurturing environment to have our babies, yet was it "safe enough" at home with a midwife?

Everyone will need to do their own homework, read the

research and books, watch the DVDs, pray, and follow their heart to know where it's best for them to give birth. For years I'd felt very strongly that home was the place, but I needed to put some fears to rest that had been planted by the society and time in which I grew up. Those fears dissipated that night, transmuted into a calm confidence that I was making the best choice for my baby and myself.

If I'd wanted to have my baby in the hospital, I still would have chosen a midwife to work as my doula. I'd want her knowledge of laboring positions and getting babies to move and get on out! That's not to say that doulas can't help immensely in that area, and doulas are usually a much more economical choice, but as anyone who knows me can attest (often with exasperation), I like to go over the top when it comes to health and getting the most natural and safe experience—whether we're talking about having a baby or just making breakfast.

At the open house I asked Selena all the questions I suggest you ask of your doula, plus a few more:

• What do you consider most important in your role as midwife?

• How do you handle a mother changing her birth plan in the middle of the birth?

- How do you handle a doctor or hospital staff member trying to encourage a laboring mother do something against her birth plan?

- Tell me a story of a birth that went perfectly.

- Tell me your most challenging birth story.

- Tell me a story of a birth that had complications and changes in plan, and how you responded.

- Do you consider twins or breach a reason to deliver in the hospital?

- In what kind of situation will you suggest a mother consider a transfer?

- In what kind of situations will you insist on a transfer?

- How long after I call and leave a message for you can I expect to hear back?

- How do you schedule your clients so you can guarantee you'll attend my birth?

- Are you planning to travel during my due date period or can you guarantee you'll be in town and available?

- Who is your backup in case you're not available, and can I have a meeting with her/them?

- What is included in your fee?

- How many prenatal and postpartum visits are included and what is involved?

- What is your refund policy if we change direction or if you and/or your partner are not available when I go into labor?

A few examples of how Selena answered my questions made me feel deeply at ease.

I asked her to tell me about something unexpected happening in labor and how she handled it. She thought a minute, laughed, and turned to her doula team. "I think she'll enjoy hearing about baby Ivan." All the doulas started to laugh warmly with the memory of what had transpired. Selena shifted in her seat and leaned forward.

There was a couple from Moscow who'd come to the U.S. during their last trimester so they could have their baby here. Perhaps citizenship issues were a factor, but top of the list for the couple was that they wanted a natural birth in which the father could participate. In Russia, medical intervention was almost 100% expected, and fathers could be seen waving to the mothers through windows from the sidewalk since they weren't allowed to be involved. That was not what they wanted, so they uprooted their lives for four months to make sure they had a magical, healthy, natural birth.

The last trimester went perfectly, the early labor went perfectly. Then when the baby was moving down the birth canal, Selena turned to her team and asked them to see if they could help determine what was going on—because suddenly it was not business-as-usual.

They all checked, and then checked again. Not one of them could tell what body part was presenting! Normally it would be the crown of the head, but sometimes the feet, bum, or some other part of the baby's body comes down the canal first. Yet with all their talent and experience, they simply had no idea what body part they'd see first.

However, with everything else stable and according to plan, Selena said they decided, "Whatever it is, this baby is doing fine, the mom is fine, and we're having this baby right here."

Shortly, a big beautiful baby was born, testicles first!

They predicted great accomplishments for a young man with that approach to life.

While it's a funny and endearing story, it's revealing.

A midwife with less experience might have panicked with a development she couldn't explain or assess, and what turned out to be a perfect birth (the testicle was a bit bruised, as the part that presents can sometimes be, but back to normal in a few days) could have been turned into a scary ambulance ride to the ER—and who knows what else.

I then asked her to tell me a story of a mother she'd accepted as a client who'd been refused by other midwives for being "high-risk." Again, she turned to her assistants and they all laughed, knowing which story she was going to tell before she started.

"Last week we had a mother give birth here at the center. She was about 5' tall and 95 pounds before she was pregnant—with twins.

"She'd been turned away by other midwives concerned for a tiny woman carrying twins. Women have been giving birth to twins," Selena commented, "since women have been giving birth, and they weren't all Amazons!"

She described the woman standing with her hands up in fists as she was crowning, pushing out both babies all by herself.

That story was reassuring and simultaneously terrifying! I believed I could squat holding onto something, or maybe give birth in a tub. But the visual of a woman standing in a mega-squat all by her tiny-self and birthing twins… wow!

Selena also told a few stories in which unexpected developments required a transfer. However, the majority of those few transfers were because the mother—originally committed to a drug-free experience—asked to go to the hospital when the pain increased.

As with the majority of births, I did have a small complication during labor that gave me a brief scare in an otherwise perfect birth. At one point a couple of hours into labor, my body—not me—started to push. Selena told me, "Allie, you're not ready yet. You're about five centimeters—don't push yet."

My eyes bulged as another contraction started and my body was jackknifing with a huge push. "It's not *me* doing it! I have no choice!"

She helped me out of the tub so she could check what was happening.

She and the doula team inspected, and as best as I can recall, apparently my uterus was tilted and the cervix opening wasn't perfectly lined up with the birth canal... or something like that! They explained that they were going to need to adjust things manually.

That was hardly a pain-free experience, but my greatest concern was if I could continue. I turned to Selena with tears in my eyes and asked: "Can I do this?"

Stone-faced, but with all the love in the world, she looked intensely into my eyes and said, *Yes!*

After they'd rearranged things and I threw up, they announced that we were through the transition; I'd gone from 5 to 10 cm and was now allowed to push—as if I'd had a choice. I hear that some women have to choose to do all the pushing that happens. When I was crowning, I had to consciously contribute to the effort, but my body knew what to do and was doing it whether or not I was onboard.

For a less experienced midwife, that might have been an overwhelming situation requiring a transfer. As it was, in her caring and strong hands my baby was born one hour later.

But our time with our midwife team wasn't over. We had several at-home appointments and our final six-week appointment with Selena was in her birth center. Until then my baby and I had hardly left the warmth of our house and sunshine of our garden. She'd never been on the highway. This appointment was our first major outing, and I was a little zealous in my care.

I hovered over our spare-no-expense, top-of-the-line mini-tank baby car seat purchased in lieu of a real tank (which are hard to find in our neighborhood). Every time my husband—sweating by now—signaled a lane change, I'd wrench my neck around to confirm we had clearance for a half-mile in all directions. During the whole drive I visualized our need to cross the busy street from the parking lot and plotted how we would do it.

When we walked in the door, Selena took one look at us. "You look stiff. What's up?"

I told her I was fine, just wound up from our first time on an eight-lane freeway moving 65 miles-per-hour.

She smiled and laughed in a way that said, *I understand, baby… let Mama kiss it and make it better.*

She asked, "Can you move?"

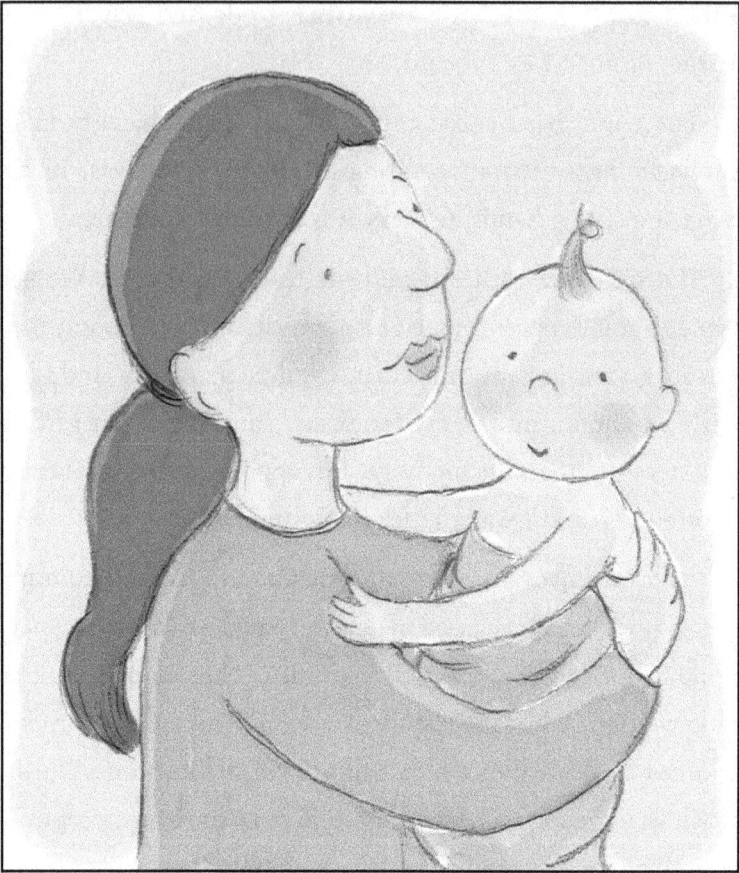

My midwife had a heart-to-heart conversation with my baby at our six-week postpartum visit, telling her she was a special person, and that it was an honor to have participated in her birth.

I looked at her puzzled. "Yes."

"Can you dance?"

"You know I can," I laughed.

"Let me see. Dance!"

While I danced (now breathing freely and blood flowing back to my face), she took Celestine to weigh and measure her, and to have a heart-to-heart talk.

Yes, to have a conversation!

When I joined them, they were hugging and looking into each other's eyes. The last bit of conversation I caught was, "... and you're a very special person. I'm so honored I got to be a part of your birth."

Ask around. That's not exactly the norm for mothers' postpartum visits with their care providers.

And yes indeed! I found my magical midwife. It made all the difference.

Visualize your perfect birth, and find your perfect help to make it happen!

THE GESTATIONAL DIABETES TEST: IS IT NECESSARY?

Do I need to take the glucose tolerance test? If I get a high score, do I need to take insulin?

For me the answer was no, and no! And here's the story...

- 50 grams of glucose
- Tap water
- Artificial food coloring

Not ingredients you'd expect to find on a "recommended" list for pregnant mothers.

Women who are discerning with the things they consume during pregnancy—or at any time in their life—are not likely going to drink the glucose test beverage without at least asking if it's really necessary.

When I was pregnant, I told my OB-GYN that I wanted to do only the most urgent testing and screening, and only if there were something that could be done to improve the situation. In other words, no tests that involved a higher risk from the test than from the problem being tested for. And certainly nothing for which the only solution offered to me would be an abortion.

She appeared to listen to my request. She said there were only about five tests that I should absolutely take. I would need to fast for 12 hours, then they would draw a few vials of blood. At the lab the next day they drew my blood, then handed me an ice-cold beverage to consume within five minutes (TCM and Ayurveda both advise not to consume extremely cold food or beverages). My doctor hadn't mentioned a test involving a drink. The ingredient list shocked me. I said there must be some mistake—this couldn't be a beverage for a pregnant woman. I wouldn't drink it at any time, much less expose my baby to those ingredients.

The lab tech insisted that it was extremely important for the baby and that my doctor said I needed it. In hindsight I am disappointed that I was susceptible to this influence, but I forgave myself, understanding that pregnant women are especially sensitive to suggestions that are offered "to protect" their baby.

I drank the liquid and immediately felt ill. I've neither slammed a freezing drink like that, nor consumed 50g of glucose in my life, even on a full stomach. I do not eat any processed foods, chemicals, or extracted sugars. (As you may now have ascertained, this means that I make almost every meal at home— from scratch.)

My test score came back high, a borderline "Failure." I was advised that I would need to go the hospital to take the next step, a 100g glucose test. (My thought was, *of course—it's like giving two freezing cold beers to down in five minutes to someone who never drinks alcohol and asking them an hour later how they feel.*) I was advised that I would need to stay in the hospital for several hours, in case I went into a coma during the test!

All the alarms went off that time.

I asked my doctor if I could simply continue to eat whole foods which do not cause glucose spikes, regularly test my own blood sugar levels with a home-test kit, and if the numbers were good, then there was indeed no problem and no need for further testing. She replied simply: "No. If you want your insurance to pay, you have to take the second test."

I researched online and found hundreds of women all with the same questions and concerns, but none clear on what to do about it.

I called my (first) midwife, who confirmed that I would need to take the second test.

I did not figure out the next step in dealing with the glucose test that day, but it was immediately clear that it was time to find a new doctor and a new midwife.

I decided to go it alone. I bought the test kit, ate my normal meals, and tested my glucose levels. All fell in the normal range!

When I finally found a doctor who genuinely respected my approach to pregnancy and nutrition, I showed him my glucose level test log. He said, "My patients, even the ones who aren't pregnant, would kill for these numbers." My new midwife: ditto.

This was the confirmation of what I already knew. I wish I'd never doubted.

My new doctor did go on to explain that the industry felt that many people would "cheat" or "lie" about their numbers if they were left to test themselves, so they had to encourage these lab tests. When women failed the tests, they were generally not trusted to change their eating habits, so to protect the mother and baby, doctors would then recommend insulin.

Fair enough.

But for mothers who are willing to control what they eat, who do not want to expose their baby to glucose rushes and chemicals, do not want to take insulin, and whose diet indeed maintains proper glucose levels, there is an answer—or at least there was for me.

My approach may not be the correct approach for all, but at least along with all the confusion and questions about the test one finds in the "pregnant community," there is an answer from someone who experienced it, found a different answer, and at 42 years of age, gave birth at home to a healthy 7lb 14oz baby.

A few tips I found important in meal preparation:

• Include protein and a small handful of nuts when eating complex carbs

• Simple carbs will cause spikes

• Flour and pasta—even whole grain—will cause higher numbers. Ideally stick to eating whole grains rather than those processed in any way

• Eat smaller, more frequent meals

• If you do eat whole grain flour products, add whole grains to the mix like whole wheat bread with cooked amaranth, quinoa, whole oats, millet, etc.

• Brown rice, yams, cherries, and berries are some of the healthiest carb sources

I appreciate that gestational diabetes can be a serious matter and must be tended to. But just as with birth choices, there are different answers for different people. No matter what the situation, if you do not feel comfortable, ask and ask again. One person saying "you must," "urgent," or "for your baby's protection" doesn't necessarily mean it is so.

Part 2:

❖ ❖ ❖

Postpartum

CHAPTER FOUR

Why Do We Need a Postpartum Doula?

T he general public in the United States is still relatively
unaware of the role and benefits of a midwife or doula.
A postpartum doula, the servant with whom we spend
the most time and who can change the course of our entire
postpartum year—and thereafter—is even less appreciated.

If this is your first birth, unless you have a loving, patient,
cool-headed mother, sister, or auntie whom you adore and who
will serve you hand and foot (and as much as we love them, this
is rare), please, sister, please... *get yourself a postpartum doula!*

If you already have children, and thus have postpartum
experience, you can imagine the benefit of qualified,
knowledgeable help from someone on your payroll.

We spend several hours on a few occasions, and then a full

day with our midwife. Ditto for our doulas. We spend anywhere from a few hours to a full day and/or night, for weeks or even a few months, with our postpartum doula.

The Chinese call the postpartum period a "sitting moon." Based on the lunar calendar, this implies that a woman should rest for a full month. By rest, they mean staying in bed with your baby—nursing, eating, and sleeping, getting out of bed only a few minutes a day for minimal grooming, a sitz bath, and using the bathroom.

Practiced for centuries, the Chinese sitting moon tradition is a complete approach to healing and bonding for mother and baby, and includes a very specific diet plan to encourage healing and abundant milk supply.

According to the precepts of Traditional Chinese Medicine, how a woman tends to her health in this short time frame is so critical that it can dictate her health and vitality in the coming years, through menopause, and beyond.

Sitting Moon, A Guide to Natural Rejuvenation After Pregnancy by Dr. Daoshing Ni and Jessica Chen is most thorough and helpful. I wrote a review for the ***Holistic Networker*** magazine, which I include at the end of Chapter 5 for those curious to learn more.

In Indian heritage, as well as Muslim and many other traditions, the time for this rest, practice, and special diet is forty days. This is not considered a luxury or only for those women with servants. It is a vital observance, an expected part of the process of having a baby.

The women I know in the U.S. rested for two or three days (if that!), and then it was more or less business as usual. To make up for the time "lost" in nursing and caring for the infant, meals—even if the mother ate well before the baby was born—are reduced to take-out and frozen dinners. The house is a disaster, mom rarely grooms, and dad swings from a helpful participant to a despondent, abandoned grouch. Desperately sad is the new trend that my cousin calls The Texas Tuck: "A few months after delivering, or even right after she has her "C," mom gets a tummy tuck and a boob job."

"That's morbid! Women can't really do that to themselves, postpartum—or ever!" I screeched.

He assured me they do. I suppose I knew that, but just didn't want to believe it.

Just like the labor and delivery practices, the postpartum period for American women has lost all the beauty and healing it can offer.

Do all women really want to know about the health effects of postpartum care or lack thereof? Probably not, but even those who don't will still be busy, overwhelmed, and tired like never before. The health of the baby and mother aside, we all need some help just to get through the period of the greatest change in our lives.

A lot of us aren't used to asking for, needing, or even liking help. We *offer* help so many times throughout our adult lives. This is the time to *ask* for the help we need. Make no mistake… you *will* need help.

What about your husband? Can't he help?

Oh, boy! (And I do mean *boy*.)

Men, God love them, are not the mothers for a reason. When they lose one or two nights of good sleep, you'd think the sky fell. Not that we don't love them, not that they don't work hard for us… but they do not—nor will they ever—understand what their partner is going through. I'm talking about the emotional shift as well as physical changes in her body, and what she needs.

Men are likely to be having their own emotional turmoil—euphoria over the birth, stress and joy over the responsibility for their new son or daughter, and dejection about no longer being the primary recipient of your time, love, and physical affection. At best, they are very helpful but a little bent. At worst, they revert to two-year-old temper tantrums and stew over losing their position as Number One at your breast!

New parenthood is a joyous and challenging learning process for *both* parents, so men should not be providing our primary postpartum care. That is the job of a woman who is multi-skilled, nurturing, not overwhelmed by the learning process, and gets a good night's sleep every night!

CHAPTER FIVE

The Role of a Postpartum Doula and How to Find One

J ust as with the relationship of a mother and her birth doula, the mother and the postpartum doula together determine the scope of the job. Pay will vary depending on the job specifics and the skills and qualifications of the postpartum doula.

Some mothers want only a few hours a day for someone to watch her baby while she rests, showers, or eats. Other women want more guidance—help with breastfeeding, soothing the baby, infant care, and support in her physical recovery (preparing sitz baths, massage, aromatherapy, etc.).

Unfortunately, I learned the list of skills I would appreciate the hard way. I was utterly clueless when I hired my postpartum doula, then deeply disappointed in her work at a time when I needed the most help. Loved my midwife, loved my doulas, loved my maid and nanny, but my postpartum doula…? A flop. Four out of five ain't bad. With help of this book, hopefully you will be thrilled with all the help involved in your birth experience and your new life as a parent.

Since my list of desired skills and capabilities may be longer than most—I look for excellence and diverse talents—I've included what I would look for. You can choose and add the skills that are a priority for you.

RAPPORT / COMMUNICATION SKILLS

This is where you ask yourself:

- How do I feel when I'm talking to this person? Do I feel she is kind, confident, knowledgeable, and a clear communicator?
- Is she listening to and supporting my ideas for postpartum or does she seem to have her own agenda?
- Would I want her around when I'm tired or frustrated?
- Most basic: Do I like her?

PHILOSOPHY / APPROACH TO POSTPARTUM CARE

Some mothers prefer a traditional approach to postpartum along the lines of a Sitting Moon. Others want to get back to "business as usual" as soon as possible. Discuss this with the postpartum doula to determine if her ideas and approach match yours.

BASIC BUSINESS SKILLS

Just because a doula comes to your home instead of a fancy corner office to work, doesn't mean she can sidestep basic business etiquette.

- Did your doula respond promptly to your initial calls?

- Is she punctual for meetings?

- Does she follow up by sending the information, contacts, and/or paperwork discussed during phone calls or meetings—without being prompted?

- Has she asked you for an outline of your philosophy and needs, and provided an outline of her philosophy and skills? Many mothers won't know what they don't know, so a postpartum doula should be able to suggest the services you are likely to need or want postpartum. You can accept or decline the various services and talents the doula offers.

SKILLS / HELP FOR THE MOTHER

Breastfeeding Support

For some mothers and babies, breastfeeding happens immediately, and as naturally as breathing. Even then, moms will often have questions. Little refinements here and there can make the experience even better.

However, many first-time mothers won't have much experience observing breastfeeding up close and personal. They may feel uncomfortable or it may not happen so naturally for emotional, physical, or other reasons. Those moms may need additional support. A doula should be able to guide a new mother through simple questions or problems. If she is a certified lactation consultant, she will have a lot of expertise and skills to get things "flowing."

Nursing is the most primal and basic action for a newborn. They want, and are often able, to latch within minutes of birth. But that's not always the case. Babies who are born into a calm, warm atmosphere and placed on their mother's chest immediately after birth have a greater chance for nature to take its course. But if the baby has drugs in its system that were given to the mother during labor—or if the baby is immediately taken from the mother and subject to multiple procedures—fear and disorientation can affect the baby's ability to latch instantly.

My postpartum doula (we'll call her Lizzy—a cute name with an *apropos* similarity to dizzy) said she'd never worked for a mother who had a drug-free birth. She was stunned at the level of awareness and connectedness she saw in my baby during her first few days after birth.

(Is it strange that I had a postpartum doula who'd never attended a woman in a home birth? Indeed! See what I mean when I say moms don't know what they don't know? Now I know that it's vital to work with a doula with experience serving in a way congruent with your desires and philosophy.)

Certainly, one can always attribute smooth breastfeeding to

blessings of good fortune, but there is plenty of evidence that supports natural birth as one way to help breastfeeding get off to a good start.

If a baby has trouble latching, and more serious issues aren't the cause, it can be resolved with the mother's patient and persistent effort, guided by a qualified lactation consultant.

Even mothers who have no trouble breastfeeding can use tips and pointers for different positions, breast care, etc. It is an important matter that will come up with almost every new mom, so a woman serious in her profession as postpartum doula should consider training as a lactation consultant to be an essential element of her service. If not, she should at the very least have contacts with local lactation experts and arrange an appointment for you.

Postpartum Massage

According to almost all schools of thought and medicine, a postpartum mother should keep physical strain to a minimum for the first six weeks postpartum while she is still bleeding (i.e., healing). Her body has been through the greatest change and expansion and contraction she will experience in her lifetime, and rest is of utmost importance.

However, bed rest often means sore spots, tight muscles, and poor circulation, which isn't conducive to healing. Massage can help in many ways. Touch is always relaxing and soothing. It helps blood and lymph circulate—thus speeding the process of healing—and it can help the little sleep mom does get come more easily.

Lizzy was so lacking in skills (including massage) that when I wanted help on short notice, I had to call Daisy, one of my birth doulas, who was certified in postpartum massage. She came immediately, and while my baby lay tucked at my side, she gave me a wonderful massage. My baby and I both fell asleep! We repeated that every day for several days. Daisy also showed me some very basic massage strokes I could do for my baby after her bath, just before bedtime.

Not all postpartum doulas will have these same skills and experience, but the kind of attention and care I received from Daisy is what you should expect. One benefit of massage I hadn't previously considered was the conversation that can arise before, during or after your massage. Daisy had so many beautiful things to share as a mother herself while caring for my body.

Some people may not want to talk, but many new moms—previously working or social butterflies—often spend more time alone with their babies than they've ever spent alone in their lives. Enjoying the brief company of another adult who is a mother, and who is simultaneously caring for you and/or your baby, is a great complement to the day.

During one visit, I told Daisy I'd had a nightmare about going out and forgetting to nurse my baby. I couldn't shake it and felt guilty about the dream. She laughed and said, "Oh, that's normal! All moms have dreams like that! When I was postpartum

I dreamed I put my baby in her carrier on top of my car and drove off without putting her *inside* the car."

Suddenly, instead of feeling bad, I felt camaraderie and part of the fun called motherhood—the best rollercoaster ride in the world!

Aromatherapy and Bach Flower Essences Therapy

These two types of therapy may not be very well known, or even a part of mainstream American lifestyle, but they are delightful, non-medical, non-invasive ways to support a mother's healing and happiness postpartum.

Since Lizzy had no knowledge of these therapies, it was Selena, my midwife, who advised me on which Bach Flower Essence to use postpartum and how. I already knew which essential oils to inhale and which to use in massage and bath.

For those unfamiliar with aromatherapy or Bach Flower Essences, a quick study of a book or online information will help you determine whether you want to include these practices in your postpartum care.

Often moms get the "baby blues" from exhaustion, blood loss, and hormonal changes postpartum (we're not talking full-on postpartum depression—that's a different subject, not addressed here). Going through this often challenging time with a multi-faceted and loving approach can help avoid or at least minimize these emotions.

Picture the difference:

Mother 1: After the first week postpartum, dad's back at work. The mother-in-law, although well-meaning, is driving the mother crackers. Mom has been essentially alone in her new world, with a body that still looks pregnant. She's bleeding, she's not sleeping, and no one is even cooking for her (the mother-in-law is microwaving a little this-and-that for her). She hasn't been touched, she hasn't left the house, and she's desperately—with her one ounce of energy—trying to be the best mom in the world to her new angel.

Mother 2: The first day postpartum, her postpartum doula arrives, prepares a warm organic sitz bath, and cares for the baby so the mother can relax and take her time in the bathroom. When mom comes out, she feels refreshed as she enters her tidied room—which smells of citrus and ginger (aromatherapy spritzer). Clean sheets await her.

She lies down and is massaged with warm oil lightly infused with lavender. After her massage, she has time with the baby while the doula either cooks or heats a warm, nourishing meal. While the mother eats, the doula either sits with her, chatting about how things are going, or she straightens the house.

You get the idea. Mother 1's story is a little depressing! Mother 2's story sounds enticing. But wait! There's more a postpartum doula could offer.

Movement and Exercise

Though her doula does not need to be a yoga teacher or physical therapist, there are a few basic stretches and movements a mother should do postpartum, especially to keep her shoulders and back free from the knots which can develop from hours of breastfeeding), and there are movements she should certainly avoid to minimize her bleeding. The doula might have a DVD or two for mom to watch, or recommend a local instructor who specializes in postpartum exercise.

Sitz Bath

A postpartum doula should know how to blend and prepare herbs for a sitz bath, because it is so soothing as well as healing every time you go to the bathroom. She should teach a mother the different ways to use the sitz: a shallow bath in the tub; a bath made to rest on the toilet seat (ideal); to use with a peri-bottle when urinating; frozen pads soaked in the infusion to use in the first few days postpartum to reduce pain and swelling.

A mother only needs to urinate one time postpartum without a peri-bottle to appreciate the need for sitz herbs! And few things will feel as good postpartum as your frozen maxi-pad that's been soaked in sitz herbs!

There are countless herbal blends for a sitz bath, but my favorite is:

Equal parts: calendula flowers, chamomile flowers,

marshmallow, rosemary, uva ursi, comfrey, and shepherd's purse, mixed with a sprinkle of lavender flowers and rose petals, and a cup of sea salt.

Forget little bags of store-bought, pre-made powder that you pour in boiling water. No matter what recipe you use, you most certainly want to use whole, fresh herbs in this preparation.

When Daisy came to give me a postpartum massage during those first few days, she saw my sitz bath "seat," meant for use on the toilet, sitting in the bathtub. She asked, "You had your sitz bath already today?"

I told her I hadn't prepared it yet.

"What's your doula doing?" She didn't wait for an answer. "Where's your sitz blend?"

I told her I had a week's worth prepared in daily portions in the freezer. She prepared my sitz bath for me while she set up for the massage.

Daisy worked professionally as an assistant midwife, lactation consultant, and birth doula—in other words, had skills far in excess of what a postpartum doula requires. However, it was not "below her" to prepare my sitz, massage me and my baby, and fold the laundry she found getting wrinkled in the dryer— all without my asking. It was so easy for her to do, but I felt like royalty—as a postpartum servant should strive to make her clients feel.

I think Lizzy was in the kitchen working out how to slice a mango at the time.

Music / Meditation

A few minutes of calm each day, listening to a guided meditation or soothing music can make all the difference for a postpartum mom. She might have her own playlist in mind, but a postpartum doula should have a recommended list of music and meditation tracks specifically for healing, recovery, and relaxation/sleep.

Recommended Reading

A postpartum doula should have a list of classic and favorite books on many subjects for the postpartum mom, including sleep training methods, co-sleeping, diaper choices, nursing, weaning, first solids, child development, newborn care, baby sign language, and mental and physical health care for the postpartum mom.

Nutrition and Meal Preparation

Knowing that no one would have the knowledge or desire to prepare the meals I would want postpartum (primarily the recipes found in the book *Sitting Moon: A Guide to Natural Rejuvenation After Pregnancy*), I bought an extra freezer and spent three months making every breakfast, lunch, and dinner I would need for the first 30 days postpartum.

Short of that, a postpartum doula should know the basic foods that are highly recommended or that should be avoided for this time. Her philosophy and attitude should align with the mother's, and she should be able to prepare at least some meals.

The ideal postpartum doula should have a strong understanding of or certification in Western Medicine, Traditional Chinese Medicine, and/or Ayurveda nutrition—and more specifically, in those aspects of each practice that address the postpartum period.

She should also know professionals in these fields to refer to for special herbs and/or recommendations, and should consult with the mother regarding her culinary and nutritional preferences. That's the Princess and the Pea approach.

Sad Lizzy's list of services written in her contract included "light cooking." Since "cooking" is a word open to infinite interpretation, this subject should be discussed at length with your doula. For Lizzy it was slicing cheese and putting crackers and apple slices on a plate. Give me a week and I could have trained my dog to bring me crackers (he's a smart boy). She had no idea, from either a Western or Eastern school of thought, about nutrition.

In addition to a list of skills, a postpartum doula should have intuition and a deep desire to help—to serve—as Daisy did.

SKILLS / HELP FOR THE BABY

Infant CPR

It is a good idea for anyone who will spend a good amount of time with your baby, including mom and dad, to be certified in infant CPR and to know the steps to take in case of an emergency.

My husband and I both took an infant CPR class taught by a firefighter/paramedic. You might feel uneasy and even ill (like me) during certain parts of the lectures, but it is invaluable training that you'll likely never need but be glad to have.

Most postpartum doulas are certified and this would be something to ask for and expect.

Infant Care

The smallest, most natural, and common phenomenon can terrify a postpartum mother.

I have a friend who was hysterical because her baby's umbilical cord fell off in four days. She'd been told it would take 2-4 weeks, so she was sure something was *terribly* wrong, even though there was no bleeding and no infection (it was fine).

Another friend called her doctor in a panic when her baby developed blisters on his lips at about two weeks (common in the early days of nursing).

My cousin didn't know if she should get her child's cradle cap wet (yes, you can).

My neighbor was scared when her baby got the first sign of a rash (many rashes, in all places, are common in newborns).

My male colleague had to call for help the first time his wife left him to change his baby's diaper: how to wipe, with what, what lotion to put on, how tightly to put on the new diaper! (Different answers for different people. The simplest is to clean very gently with a wash cloth and water, dry thoroughly, and either no lotion or cream or perhaps a little coconut oil.)

Few new moms know that when an infant falls asleep in your arms, you should place him bottom down first, and then slowly lower the back, neck, and head last (babies wake up if you let their head touch the surface of the bed first).

I didn't know what to do about my newborn's earwax! (Most common answer: nothing. Leave it alone.) As a new mom or dad, every new appearance, sound, or action is a potential cause for joy or alarm.

A doula should verse the parents on all basic infant care—including bathing, diaper changing, body care, and grooming. Parents can relax (though not entirely), knowing that their postpartum doula is extremely experienced, has seen it all, and will be able to guide them in this completely natural but utterly foreign journey of the first month(s) of parenthood.

Swaddling

There are varying schools of thought, but it is an old and common practice around the world, and newly accepted in the U.S. as a standard practice, to swaddle babies for sleep the first three months postpartum (often referred to as the "fourth trimester").

A doula should know the benefits of swaddling, as well as the various methods and products used for swaddling. She should teach the parents how to wrap their baby if they want to swaddle their little one—which is best determined ahead of time.

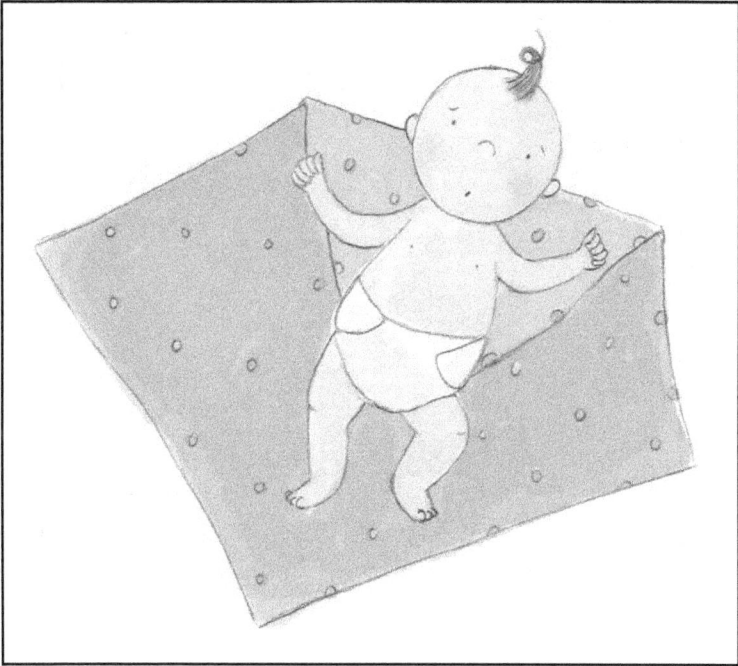

Baby unswaddled

Bassinette, Crib, and Co-sleeping

Before the birth, the postpartum doula should help parents decide where the baby will sleep. She should help them understand the impacts and needs that come with each option.

If a doula is very strongly opposed to the newborn sleeping in a crib in a separate room, and the parents have chosen that method, that may be a significant enough disconnect in philosophies to merit looking for another doula. With such an important issue, parents and postpartum caretakers should be on the same page.

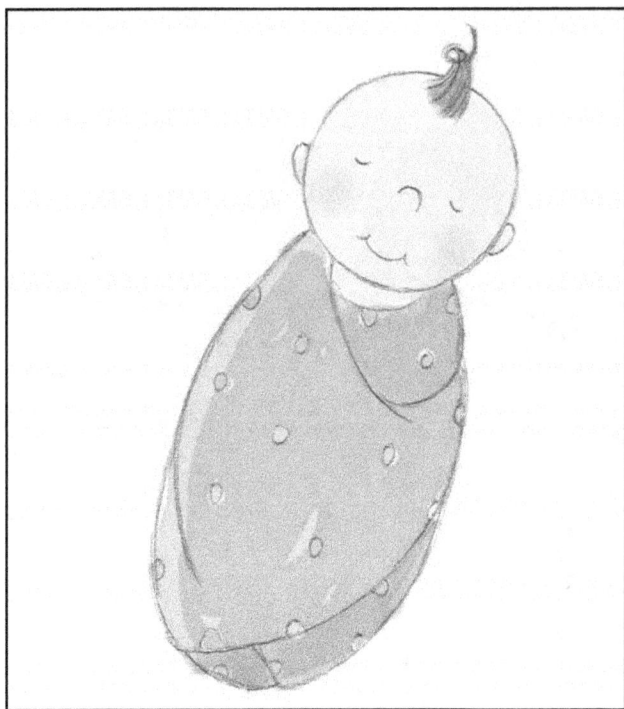

Baby swaddled

No matter how experienced and wise a postpartum doula may be, or how informed or clueless new parents may seem, beliefs and agendas cannot be pushed from either side.

On-demand vs. Scheduled

Many parents feel most comfortable allowing their infants to nurse and sleep according to their timing and desire—hence the name, on-demand.

Others feel it is better to get babies accustomed to a nursing and sleeping routine, determined by the parents, at a very early age. This inevitably leads to a cry or no-cry method approach to parenting—a very touchy subject, indeed.

There is much research supporting the wisdom of each approach, and a postpartum doula should be familiar with each philosophy, recommend books for the parents to read before the birth (if they haven't already decided on an approach) and support the parents in the approach they decide is best.

Diapers and Diaper Rash

A doula should know about regular ol' plastic disposable diapers, "green" disposable diapers, cloth diapers, and local diaper services—and be able to support the mother in making a decision about how to diaper her baby.

She should also counsel the parents on the ways to avoid diaper rash: coconut oil as a natural diaper cream, changing frequently (even at night), and some "buns in the sun" time rather than leaving baby's bottom sealed up all day and night.

Getting Baby Around: Baby Carriers/Wraps/Strollers/Car Seats

There are countless choices for transporting baby. With dozens of ways to "wear" a baby and countless strollers and car seats, a postpartum doula can help guide parents' decisions by determining their priorities: comfort, contact, safety, expense, durability, convenience, weight, ease of set-up, etc.

When I was a few days postpartum, Lizzy recommended a wrap that distributed the weight of the baby primarily around the waistline by wrapping several times tightly around the midriff. The first time I used it, I had an immediate increase in postpartum bleeding—and was discouraged from using a carrier. It was an excellent wrap, but best used several weeks to months after the baby is born.

There are other carriers that distribute the weight over the mother's shoulders and back. They are more appropriate when the baby is small (and won't put a strain on the mother's back) and when mom doesn't need extra pressure on her abdomen.

There are many well-designed car seat systems: some rotate to more easily situate the baby, some detach from a base to set on a stroller base, etc. Each option must be considered, then parents should practice—with guidance—placing their baby in the carriers or seats before actually needing to do so.

Finally, many people fail to install their car seats properly— it's not as easy as clicking a seat belt.

A postpartum doula can help a parent with installation, but she should know where to send the parent to have the installation checked by someone qualified—the fire department, the highway patrol or maybe an AAA office, depending on your city.

Infant Massage

Infant massage is not considered a luxury in many cultures. In India, for example, it is considered an essential and joyful part of the daily grooming and care for an infant.

For anyone interested in the subject, it is fascinating, highly beneficial, and fun for babies. Mothers can learn basic infant massage techniques from reading a book or two, including what organic food-source oils are best for babies' skin and appropriate to your climate.

Certification and extensive experience in infant massage is another talent a committed and health-conscious postpartum doula would likely offer.

ADDITIONAL SKILLS / HELP FOR THE FAMILY

Driving

If parents are going to ask a postpartum doula to drive their older children to school (I wouldn't leave my children alone in the care of a servant, but many people do), they should run a background check (in addition to calling the doula's references). The postpartum doula should have a recent copy of her driving record from the Department of Motor Vehicles, a current insurance card, and a functioning, appropriate vehicle.

Errands

A postpartum doula should establish a routine with the mother in which they decide, for example, that the doula will send a text or call when she's on the way each day, to see what errands she can run or things she can pick up for the family.

It's good to have an understanding that if the mother doesn't respond within 15 minutes, the doula will know that nothing is required that day and she can drive straight to work. This eliminates the mother's need to watch for the call and to respond if she doesn't need anything.

Community Connections and Network

For any talent or skill listed above in which the postpartum doula is not certified or qualified, she should have a local network of people who can perform those services.

The last thing a woman in her third trimester or already postpartum needs is to research names, check referrals, conduct interviews, and so on for every service she needs. That's the work that whole HR departments are assigned.

Nor should she experiment by hiring whomever she can find and going through waves of people to get to the right one. (I assure you it is not something you want to experience postpartum. You want to focus on your joyful bundle!)

As I've mentioned enough times, Lizzy was not a qualified

postpartum doula. So how did I, with this list of the services I would look for and require, end up with her? As I said earlier: you don't know what you don't know—until you've been through it—and you don't know what your servants *should* know. But now I do—and so do *you*!

I hadn't even heard of a postpartum doula before I was pregnant. I met Lizzy at a clothing store for babies when I was about seven months pregnant. She was sweet, polite, and came highly referred.

The first sign that she was not going to be up to snuff was when I called her after having my baby—and didn't hear back for 24 hours. As with the first midwife I engaged and quickly disengaged, Lizzy was kind but she did not approach her work as a business. Thinking it was acceptable to be camping in a "no-signal" zone for two days, she left her clients wondering what happened to her for an entire weekend.

Simply unacceptable!

However, I was one day postpartum—and that's not the time to look for different help. But after about a week of her "help," and Daisy's repeatedly shaking her head in disgust as she did the work the postpartum doula should have done (while she was there officially just to give me a massage), I figured out that I needed someone else and set out to find that person.

WHAT DO POSTPARTUM DOULA SERVICES COST?

If a postpartum doula were to have the complete list of qualifications outlined in this chapter, she could easily command $10,000 for working full days in a 30-40 day postpartum sitting moon engagement.

Doing the math for the individual services, daily in-house massages for mom and baby alone are worth $100 each (times 30-40 days).

This complete list of skills would take years of dedicated work to acquire, and a person with that level of dedication and achievement would have innate abilities that are hard to find in most people. Further, if a person did have this complete list of qualifications, they would be in high demand amongst a crowd that can easily afford and demand that level of service.

For most of us, the complete list is not necessary and wouldn't fit our budget. The good news is, there are a lot more postpartum doulas who do not have even close to that complete list of skills, yet are very good in at least a few of them. In that instance, they would likely command $30-$40 per hour.

Moving down the line, a doula who is kind, professional, dependable, and has just one or two of those skills would command $20-$30 per hour.

Next, people who are just great at holding babies and letting mom have a shower or nap should not be calling themselves doulas (though they do). They are, in fact, babysitters, and are doing less than I did as a babysitter at twelve. $10-$12 per hour is generous.

Finally, people like Lizzy, kind and well-intentioned but without skills or business sense, should stop inflicting themselves on innocent, unknowing mothers until they can get some training. She might have potential. I hope she's in a class right now.

BOOK REVIEW & AUTHOR INTERVIEW
SITTING MOON:
A Guide to Natural Rejuvenation After Pregnancy

As originally published in the Holistic Networker, Winter 2011 Issue

How does a woman quickly and safely rejuvenate after childbirth, provide well for her baby, get back to her old energy level, and back into her old jeans? Have a sitting moon!

Sitting Moon?

In use for thousands of years, the Chinese calendar is a lunisolar calendar, indicating the phase of the moon. According to Traditional Chinese Medicine (TCM), to rejuvenate after childbirth a woman should rest for approximately one month, or one "moon."

Thus we have the title of the new book from Dr. Daoshing Ni and Jessica Chen about natural postpartum rejuvenation, **Sitting Moon**.

In a country where women are often back on their feet and running soon after giving birth, one month's rest may sound shocking, but this practice is common in many countries around the world today, and has been throughout history. The reasons are many, but the two primary purposes are to allow the mother to regain the strength and essence she gave to the baby and lost in childbirth, thus supporting her long-term vitality; and time and ability for her to deeply nurture and bond with her newborn.

In case those reasons aren't compelling enough, there is also a list of ways a woman may suffer long-term if she does not take time to heal after childbirth.

While the subject of infant care and breastfeeding are often covered extensively in books, training classes, and even some hospitals, the mother's postpartum care—if not completely ignored—certainly takes last place.

Since the mother's health and well-being support her *and* the infant in all ways, this new book has an important place in every mother's and care-provider's library.

What you'll find in the book

When I heap praise on this book, I speak from personal experience. When six months pregnant, I knew it was "now or never" to start preparing the nutritious meals I would need postpartum, so I bought a freezer and jumped on my computer to begin a search for postpartum recipes I could prepare in advance.

Unless you're comfortable eating any ol' dish someone prepares or brings from a restaurant, asking someone to search out top quality ingredients and prepare the exact three meals per day plus snacks you would prefer postpartum is likely expecting too much! Naturally postpartum moms are grateful for any help, but you get the idea here.

When I sat at the computer to commence the search, there was an auspicious email announcing the release of **Sitting Moon,** which I ordered immediately.

What I found in **Sitting Moon** was far more than a postpartum meal plan. Almost any topic of interest or need for the postpartum mother is addressed: yoni care, breast care, and natural remedies from TCM for numerous ailments of mind, body, and spirit. There are also special sections that address issues and offer recommendations for mothers recovering from a C-section, which today could mean 35-45% of all mothers giving birth in a hospital.

As it is so vital to the effectiveness of a sitting moon, approximately 2/3 of the book is dedicated to the role of nutrition in healing and producing ample milk. There are recipes offered week-by-week for the 4-week sitting moon, and they are specific for that week's rejuvenation needs. They are all surprisingly simple to prepare, most include ingredients that are readily available, and they are absolutely delicious.

Forget chicken bits in a gooey sweet and sour sauce—these recipes have titles such as: *Scallops with Broccoli, Vegetable Barley Soup, Baked Sesame Tofu,* and most adventurous, *Peanut and Pork Knuckle Soup.* There are many recipes and suggestions for vegetarian moms, as well. Many recipes do include Chinese herbs and those can be purchased from a Chinese medicine practitioner or herbalist.

As a last bit of evidence of the efficacy from my personal

experience with a sitting moon, and to further encourage mothers: as a first-time mom at 42 years old, I had a home birth, abundant milk supply, and was back in my old clothes in six weeks—all by taking a full month's rest with my baby, and eating three meals plus two snacks per day of excellent food!

Interview with *Sitting Moon* authors Dr. Daoshing Ni and Jessica Chen

I had the opportunity to speak with the authors and to inquire furher on the topic of postpartum recovery and how Chinese Medicine addresses the issues.

Q. Many women say, "I feel better and ready to move around," often as soon as 2-3 days after giving birth. How can the decision to return to an active lifestyle quickly after delivery affect a woman's health in the long run?

A. When women say they're feeling great and ready for action again after a few days, this can be the adrenaline from labor. This is viewed as "false" energy. So in actuality, your body is still recovering.

If you do not take some time to allow your body to heal it can run into problems in the future. A year down the line you may find yourself being more tired, having a difficult time sleeping, with difficulty in losing the pregnancy weight, or joint pain. In addition, the mother's body is still "open", "loose", and "tired" in the pelvic region.

Having a normal and sometimes overly active lifestyle too quickly can cause problems in the pelvic region such as bleeding disorders, hernia, or hemorrhoids.

Q. In your book, you address special issues for women over 35 or having had a C-section. IVF pregnancies are ever on the rise, even with women under 35. What special needs do they have, and would you add that category to the group who need to take special care with a Sitting Moon?

A. Care for IVF moms should fall under the category of women over 35 and C-section. The process of IVF takes a lot out of a woman; therefore it is important to bring more nourishment to their body after giving birth. Many IVF expecting mothers tend to be more emotionally tired. They will need more relaxation and personal time to heal, which is in short supply once the woman becomes a new mother. Therefore, a plan for such healing activities should be contemplated and scheduled before the labor process.

Q. It is common, and said to be "normal," that women lose a tooth with a pregnancy or lose a substantial amount of hair after childbirth. Is that to be expected or is it a sign of something that can be addressed and/or prevented?

A. It is normal to lose hair after labor due to the hair that was not shed during pregnancy. But if the hair loss is excessive, it can be a sign of lack of nutrients. According to Chinese medicine, hair is related to blood and the kidney/adrenal/reproductive system. When the blood is flowing abundantly and the kidney/adrenal/reproductive is strong, hair will be full and strong.

Naturally after childbirth, the mother is deficient in both. This issue can be prevented and addressed with acupuncture (bringing more blood flow to the head) and Chinese herbs (providing nutrients to the body). Of course, eating well and getting some shut-eye is also important.

Q. The explanations one commonly hears for postpartum depression, anxiety, and/or nightmares seem to fall short, and women are often prescribed antidepressants as the remedy. Even when women are happy with their pregnancy and adore their babies, they can experience these symptoms. Can you explain it in TCM terms and describe the approach to address these issues?

A. In TCM, mood disorders after labor can be due to depletion of blood and lack of sleep. The blood loss from the labor leads to the blood not able to nourish the heart and spirit. In TCM, the heart is one of the organs that is related to your mood. Lack of sleep can also affect your mood. Your body heals and regenerates when you sleep. When your body does not get the proper amount of rest, it does not provide the right amount of nutrients to your body and can therefore further enhance mood changes.

Q. In a breastfeeding class I audited, an attendee asked the lecturing nurse about eating spicy food and junk foods while breastfeeding. The answer provided was, "Your baby does not eat what you eat—it's different." However, if the body uses what we eat to make blood, and breast milk is made from the proteins, sugars, and fat in the mother's blood, what we eat has an immediate and direct relationship on what our baby eats. Your comments from a TCM perspective?

A. Even though the main compositions of the breast milk are fat, protein,t and carbohydrates, there are many micronutrients as well as other trace chemicals that tag along with the breast milk delivered to the baby. Therefore certain nutrients and trace chemicals, such as in spicy foods and cured meats, can still be transferred in a minute amount to the breast milk. This normally should not impact the baby adversely when eaten in a small amount.

From the TCM perspective, it is very important for the nursing mother to eat a diverse spectrum of whole foods and stay away from manufactured foods (processed and packaged foods). This way, the baby will be exposed to different nutrients and learn how to digest and absorb these nutrients.

Q. The recipes in Sitting Moon are delicious, easy to prepare, and nutrient-rich. Would you recommend those recipes for mothers beyond the first postpartum month?

A. Yes! The moms can continue to prepare these meals up to one year after delivery. They are especially good to have when the moms get their first menstrual flow after delivery. These meals are also excellent for women to have at the tail end of or after their menstrual flow.

Q. Can we look forward to more books on a related subject—*Your Baby's First Two Years: Recipes and Common Herbal Remedies,* for example? (I would vote for that.)

A. Sounds like an excellent idea! Maybe also on healthy eating during pregnancy.

Q. Thank you. We'll look for those!

Part 3:

❖ ❖ ❖

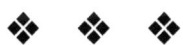

Raising an Infant

Chapter Six

Why Do We Need a Maid, Cook, or Nanny?

After reading Parts 1 and 2, you may be warming to the concept of having servants and how deeply beneficial it is for the family—and great for the servant as well. In almost any other country in the world, this has always been known (whether family members or hired servants), but in the U.S. we're still catching on.

Let's start by addressing the question: *Who doesn't need help?*

Clearly, people who live in tightknit extended families with everyone contributing time and finances to benefit the whole will not need the same amount, if any, of hired help to raise their family. It takes a village—and they've got one.

The only other group is parents who are happy living exhausted, rushed, compromised, messy, ill-fed, exercise- and sleep-deprived—who end up with kids who are ADD (attention from the parents deficit disorder) and raised primarily by advertisers via TV.

Everyone else: We need help!

My experience in this area is what compelled me to write this book. I spent 35 years working, traveling, exercising, training, pursuing interests—carrying the knowledge that when I did have a family, I would put all that aside for a few to several years, and dedicate myself completely to the care of hearth and home.

My husband and I are both immigrants to California; so neither of us has family or lifelong friends here to help us raise our children. In that scenario, servants are a must.

Back to the list of what I wanted to do, be, and offer to my family as a mother: to cook three whole food, organic meals a day from scratch. No microwave, boxes, or plastic.

I wanted to nurse my baby full-time until she and I decided we're ready to wean—one year, maybe two?

I wanted to be the primary teacher for my child, even when (or if) she attends a school, and my husband wants to be the co-primary teacher.

I wanted to kiss my husband as he walks out the door to work and have at least a little time with him when he comes home in the evening.

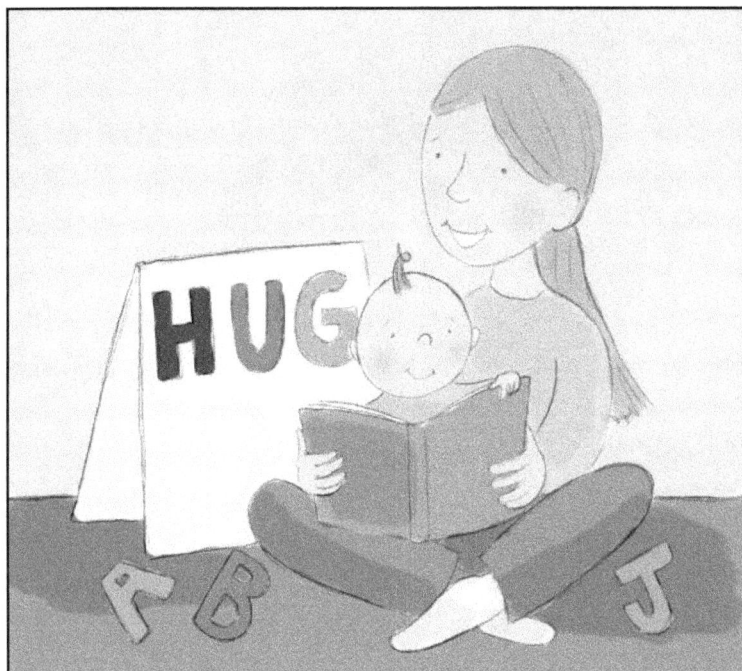

Quality help frees parents to spend time with their babies in more fun and productive ways.

I wanted our house—great or small—to be our family palace: a place that is clean, beautiful, inviting, and in which we are happy to spend our time.

My husband and I wanted time to exercise, read, and pursue other interests together.

To sum it up, I wanted to *be with my family*, not just see them in passing between the office, the drive-through window, and the bed where I would fall in a coma.

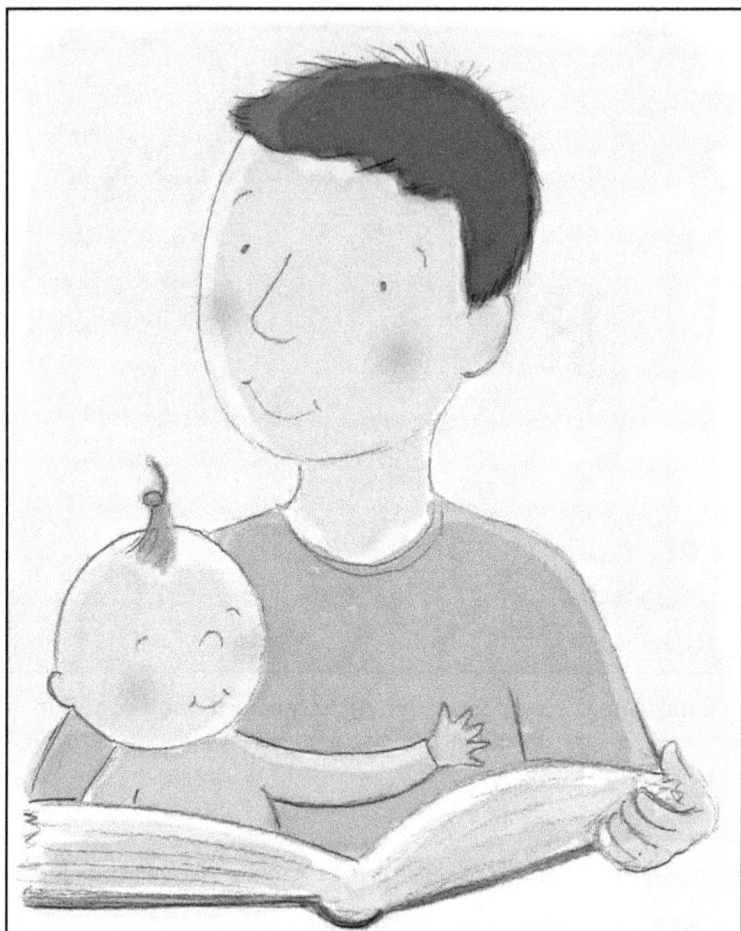

Parents are able to spend more quality time with their babies if not swamped with daily duties and chores.

One can already see that achieving all of that, with husband working all day and wife caring for baby all day and night (and perhaps also working in an office), would be impossible without help.

But what kind of help do we need, how much, what should they do, and how do we find them?

There are many kinds of servants, but the three we will focus on here are those who are the most immediate help for parents raising an infant: a maid, a cook, and a nanny.

In the U.S., we're just getting used to the idea that it is essential to have a doula, midwife, and postpartum doula. But people are familiar with the roles of maid, cook, and nanny. My premise is that people are accustomed not only to over-paying for substandard service from these three types of servants, but the servants are also primarily used to reduce the amount of time a parent spends with their child. I see their fullest potential in these roles, in a way that allows parents to be more involved, energized, healthy and hands-on with their children! This book is written for people who *want* to be with their children; who are looking for more, not less time with them; who want to feed, teach, and entertain them with high standards.

Naturally, I know a few mothers who *long* for the nanny to arrive so they can rush off to their nail, hair, luncheon and shopping appointments, and not have to hear their children's requests or have them seeking attention all day.

Yet even people who hire maids, cooks, and nannies so they can return to their independent lives, free from the dictates of their babies' schedules, can benefit from reading the following chapters.

I not-so-secretly hope that the information in the following chapters will encourage those people to spend more—not less—time with their children when they have qualified servants working for them. With qualified help, parents will feel less tired and run-down, they will have more energy and patience, till they will gradually and naturally want to spend more time with their children again.

Parents of infants should be bathing their infant together—not cleaning the floors, sinks, and toilets while baby watches TV. Moms—homemakers and *especially* working moms—should be cuddling with and reading books to their babies, not washing, chopping and cooking every fruit, vegetable, grain, legume, herb, and spice the family will eat and washing every dish used. Dads should be playing in the garden with babies or helping them sing their ABCs—not sweeping out the garage every weekend while baby watches from the distance in her playpen. Of course servants won't do *all* the housekeeping, chores, and cooking—but the point is that they *help*, allowing us to spend more quality time with our babies.

As much as we do want to be with our children every minute, it does help immensely to have someone watch the baby occasionally while we shower, cook, clean, or even—imagine—take a few minutes to exercise, read, or sit in meditation.

Lacking aunties, grandparents, and siblings in our homes helping us care for our children, it's good to have at least one other face for your child to see from time to time! And that's where our maids, cooks, and nannies come in. (This is, of course, assuming you have found an excellent servant.)

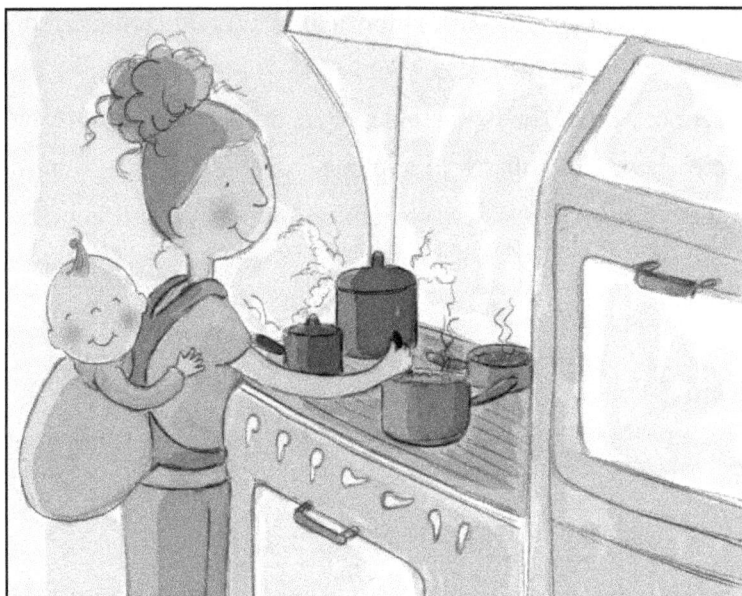

My nanny and I take turns with all the requirements of the day. For example, sometimes she cleans while I cook.

I've created an unusual scenario with my servant—I call her my personal assistant, she calls herself my house manager. She's a lot nanny, a little bit cook, and a tiny bit maid—and it works perfectly for her and my family.

Though her role is often understood as nanny, I never leave her alone with my baby. Many people have no idea what I mean when I say that or why I would want to say that. But it is the case.

I have always been uncomfortable with the thought of leaving a person—a baby—who is unable to speak, to care for or defend himself in any way, alone and at the mercy of someone

I have not known my entire life (such as a loving grandparent). That other people find it acceptable is their business, but for a lot of people around the world and for me, it is simply unthinkable. There are far too many examples of people saying, "But she seemed so nice…" or "Everyone liked him—who could imagine he would…"

No way.

Further, basic safety aside, I want to be with my baby. I want to care for her night and day. I am her mother and I want to mother her. I know I'm blessed getting to do so.

So what does my personal assistant do?

Sometimes she plays with my baby, reads to her, and helps her practice her sign language, and I watch them while I cook. Sometimes she cooks or prep-cooks while I spend time with my baby. Sometimes I pop in a yoga DVD, my baby watches me practice (and tries to imitate the poses—often doing them better than I can), and our nanny changes the sheets and does laundry.

While I'm running errands, at the park, or visiting friends, she cleans the house and I return to a fresh kitchen, empty trash cans, and carpets vacuumed in straight lines. If I need anything from the grocery store, any errand run, any phone call made… she will do it.

It's a wonderful scenario allowing me to spend the maximum amount of time with my baby and husband, to prepare and eat nutritious meals, to have at least a little "personal" time, and to have a clean house.

Everyone will have different needs, desires, and income to allocate to paying for help. Sometimes those needs can be filled by one servant working full-time, a part-time servant working just a few hours a week, or a few servants with different schedules.

In the following chapters, I outline the role of maid, cook, and nanny, and offer ideas for finding them and working out the schedule and role that works best for your family.

Don't Be Discouraged from Hiring Help Because It's "Too Expensive"

In this book I outline the expense involved with the various servants who can support bonding, healing, and growth for new parents. It is my premise that perhaps not all, but the majority of Americans, even in these times, can afford at least some help... *if that becomes their priority.*

I say this with love and empathy for those experiencing financial challenge and making tough choices. At age 13 I worked at Haagen Dazs after school so I would have money for the little extras... like food and basic toiletries. During high school, college, and a few years after graduation, I had to make frequent shifts in priorities and reallocate budget. Decisions such as: should I get a full tank of gas and skip the grocery store, or a half-tank and eat dinner tonight? Should I fix the driver's-side window of my car so it rolls up and I'm not rained on for the next six months, or should I buy text books for class this semester? I spent the last weeks of many months worrying how I was going to make rent.

Remember the Vidal Sassoon Shampoo commercials: *if you don't look good, we don't look good*. Well, in college I found gallon-size bottles of that shampoo for a few dollars and I stocked up. I'd use it to wash my hair, and for anything else that needed cleaning. As I'd pour Vidal Sassoon into the washing machine I'd smile and say, "If your clothes don't look good, we don't look good."

We're a blessed folk in this country of abundance, and many of us have become so accustomed to the countless indulgences and small luxuries we enjoy on a daily basis that we call them necessities. I know people who—though considered to be living at the very lowest income level—still have their hair done and get manicures regularly, drink expensive and unnecessary beverages (we're talking alcohol, sodas, and coffee here), buy new electronics and clothes frequently, and expend their limited budget on other non-essential items. When our priorities shift, often the things and services we deem "necessary" change and we reallocate our budgets accordingly.

At the very least, the budget can generally be found to hire a maid or nanny to help a few hours once per week for approximately $50–$75 if it is a priority. There are some people who genuinely have nothing to cut from their budget and can't afford help. I have ideas for them, too—more on that later.

CHAPTER SEVEN

The Role of a Maid and How to Find One

The best lesson I learned about being a maid myself was cleaning house for a woman named Alex who years before had made a small fortune with her own cleaning company. Her house was all white: towels, linens, furniture, appliances, counters, cabinetry, carpet, artwork, dishes, toiletries, and tissue paper... white. Not only was it white, it was also extraordinarily clean.

The first few times I cleaned for her, I couldn't imagine what she was paying me to do. I had my staff go though the motions, but it felt uncomfortable, like we were being paid for nothing. After our third visit, Alex called me on a Saturday and said we needed to meet—it was *important*. Wondering what could have happened, I agreed to drive to her house. When I arrived, she asked what I thought she'd hired me to do. I told her that was an excellent question I'd been asking myself.

She then told me the many ways in which we'd failed in our duty, some of which were:

• We didn't lift stove burners and remove the drip pans that rest under the burners so we could wipe *under* them (she demonstrated, slowly, and then peered into my eyes, looking for the shame she should find there).

• We failed to dust the top of every picture and doorframe (she ran her finger over one or two and rolled her eyes to demonstrate our weakness and her disgust).

• Why hadn't we pulled apart the rubber seal that lines the door of the fridge and freezer? If we had, we'd have found breadcrumbs (she pulled at the rubber seal vigorously, sending crumbs flying with a dramatic sweep of her arm).

• There were fingerprints on the bathroom cabinet doors (she used a police mag light to illuminate the fingerprints and asked in an alarmingly low and slow voice: "Do... you... call... that... clean?"). I could feel her simmering fury, and I began to worry for my personal safety.

But after the demonstration she calmed down and said that she'd like me to keep me on if I thought my staff could do the job properly. Those with less temerity or perhaps more intelligence would have used that time to say, "I'm afraid we're just not up to the task" and bow out.

However, I was impressed. She'd turned "clean" into a fanatical religion, a branch of the military, and a great love. If I could please her, I would have an entirely new understanding of "clean"—and I could earn anyone's business.

I learned a lot in the early days of my cleaning business. I have seen maids who work with artistry, maids who work with acceptable basic skills, and maids who should either hide at home, or—if they must inflict themselves on the public—hire on as a telephone customer service representative for a big American bank where they'll fit in well.

A maid, like any other servant, must have a personality that is pleasing, or at least harmonious with yours. And she must have the skill set you require.

Equally important, when you find someone with whom you feel a personality "click," you should also feel at least a moderate sense of trust immediately. I've learned from experience, any red flags or strange feelings in the beginning usually prove to have been valid warnings of future problems.

Here's your next useful list—the skills I require of my maids (I'm slightly more forgiving than Alex). Select from it, adding or deleting items to fit your needs as you search for help.

Punctuality:

Did the maid call you back the same day or the next morning after you first made contact? Did she arrive on time for her interview or her first time cleaning?

Being at home so much, I'm fairly flexible with my maid's schedule, but I expect people to do what they say. So if we've agreed that she's coming at 10:00 a.m. on Wednesday, it is acceptable if she wants to be an hour or two late—but she needs to call or text and notify me by 8:00 a.m.

If I worked or was frequently away from home and was changing my schedule to allow my maid into my home (assuming she doesn't have a key), I would expect absolute punctuality.

Late once negatively affects my schedule, but it happens to everyone. Late twice: on notice. Three times: find other arrangements.

References:

How many references did she offer and how quickly after you asked did she provide them? Did they sound like relatives or were these really clients? Did the referrals hesitate when they spoke, or were they happy to speak about their experience? If you left a voicemail message, did they call you back?

I would ask for three references before allowing someone in my home and around my family—even though I'm always present. In the past, whenever I failed to adhere to this rule, I regretted it.

On the flip side, when someone has done outstanding work for me and uses me as a professional reference, I always make sure to return calls to their potential client and tell them warmly about my experience.

When you call references, have a list of questions that are most important for you to know. My list is short and concise:

1.) Is she punctual, professional and dependable?

2.) Does she know her craft, or have you needed to do a lot of teaching?

3.) Is she motivated, or do you need to prod her to work?

4.) Would you trust her alone in your home and around your children?

While their answers to these questions may vary greatly from my own assessment, it is often interesting and revealing to hear what they say. For example, answering with a hesitant "Yeah" to question #4—as opposed to "she's like family"—is telling.

Appearance and attire:

Does she wear a uniform? If not, is she modest and clean in appearance?

Maids—people who clean for a living—should look, well… clean! They should not be dressed scantily or slovenly.

Most folks don't require uniforms anymore, nor do maids choose to wear them. I don't require the help in my home to wear them. That said, I like uniforms, and in my business we wore them. I think they bring respect to the individual and the industry.

In my cleaning company, the maids (and I) wore pink tennis shirts (which I purchased for them), knee-length khaki shorts, pink socks, and white tennis shoes. Our uniforms were clean, we wore our hair tied back, and everyone looked fresh and well groomed.

Who wants a maid cleaning their home in a stained concert t-shirt, daisy dukes or tattered sweat pants, and scruffy slippers or flip-flops? If a maid is professional and successful, she will have the funds to own clean, decent clothing and will take pride in wearing it to work.

Skills and knowledge:

This is a big subject, so we'll break it down, room by room. This will by no means be a thesis on the topic, which I could—and may—write at another time, but it's a sufficient outline of good and decent service.

Every maid will clean a little differently. They'll have their favorite and least-favorite tasks—and it will reflect in the job. Everyone will have days when they're bursting with energy and off-days when they blow it. Fine. In general, I expect more than they know or do, at least at first, because most of them grew up with mothers who didn't clean, or not well, and they've never had professional training.

The time in the house should be divided roughly in threes. 1/3 of the time should be in the kitchen, 1/3 the time in the bathrooms, and the remaining 1/3 dusting, vacuuming, and miscellaneous tasks. There should be a common sense approach to task order and timing, so everything is complete in the time allotted.

Let's look at a basic 3-hour shift for a 2-bedroom, 2-bath house or apartment. (You will probably want to print these directions below and hand them—as-is or amended by you—to your maid. It will be much easier than training them on every step and reminding them every time they clean.)

A 3-hour clean is "basic" because it does not allow for details such as removing all items from refrigerator and cleaning the inside, sweeping out a garage, ironing, or washing windows. It should include:

1.) Laundry—which takes approximately 30 minutes in the wash and an hour in the dryer. Therefore, if any laundry is to be done, it is started immediately.

Do not assume your maid knows how to do laundry, to use any appliance correctly, or even how to use your cleaning products. I've had almost everyone who worked for me toss my gorgeous stainless steel and copper cookware in the dishwasher, along with fine cutlery and china. These items are to be *hand* washed and dried.

I've had a maid use Windex on a cherry wood desk. When I asked her why she did that, she said that I had explained Windex was to be used on glass and shiny surfaces, and my wood desk was shiny. And I've had a proud college grad throw white hand-knit silk and wool baby clothing in the washer and dryer with reds. A professional would either know the proper way to clean or finish the task, or would at least know enough to ask your preference.

Expect to spend a good amount of time monitoring and mentoring in the first few days and weeks with any servant. After that, however, expect them to remember and perform the duties as you've discussed together.

2.) The kitchen should be cleaned next, as it can take the longest, or if done in less than one hour, allows for more intensive cleaning in the other areas. Here's a task list:

- Dishwasher emptied.
- Dirty dishes washed and put away.
- All items removed from stove and counter tops.
- Counters, sink(s), cabinets, large appliances (including the neglected, dusty top of the fridge, over the hood and sides of the oven—if they can be reached), and stove scrubbed and dried.

- All items and small appliances wiped down and returned to their proper place. Sometimes maids will return items to a different place in order to "prove" to the employer that they were removed and thoroughly cleaned. Few things are more irritating than having to "redo" your entire house after the maid has rearranged everything. But perhaps the maid just can't remember where the items were and has done her best.

I usually know which reason was the cause of the redecorating. In the first case, I politely tell them to knock it off. In the second, I gently request they pay a little more attention and try to replace things where they found them.

- Finally, the floor should be swept, mopped, and dried.

As with every room, the kitchen should be assessed after completion. Are there streaks on any of the surfaces or appliances? Crumbs missed in the corners of the counter tops or floor? Is the trashcan completely empty with a replacement liner? Is the paper towel roll almost empty and ready for a fresh roll to be put out?

If all is spotless… on to the next task.

(Around 30 minutes after they've begun, the maid should switch the laundry to the dryer, and if needed, start the next load.)

3.) Assuming the kitchen requires the full hour, the next hour is dedicated to the bathrooms:

- As with the kitchen, all items are to be removed from the countertops, sink, bathtub, shelves, and floor. This includes the soap, shampoo bottles, etc. that are in the tub or shower stall. They should be wiped down with a wet sponge, dried, and placed on a towel on the floor outside the bathroom (the toothbrush is NOT to be placed next to the toilet bowl brush, as "the college grad" did).

• The trash should be emptied and the trash can wiped down. However, if it is covered with months or years of nastiness, the owner should replace the can and not ask a servant to do something they haven't done themselves. (As demanding as I am of servants, I never ask them to do what I wouldn't do, or to make up for clients' slovenly ways.) After the trash can is wiped and dried, a fresh liner is placed inside.

My oven is clean (with a few spills). My trashcans are clean and lined. My fridge is clean and the food in it is fresh (with the occasional spill). I wipe down my bathroom sink, countertop, and mirror after each use. It takes a mere second and it maintains a minimum level of cleanliness.

In summary, I don't expect my maids to have HAZMAT gear and training! If a house does require HAZMAT intervention, well, one doesn't ask a professional servant to do that revolting work. A pro would flee a house of horrors and save their talent for people who care for their property and dwelling.

When I owned my cleaning company, I made one exception to the HAZMAT rule. If the person for whom we were cleaning was elderly and alone, I viewed that person as a dear grandparent unable to care properly for him or herself, so I would clean the messes personally. My maids appreciated and respected that, and they were all the more willing to do the borderline HAZMAT jobs we encountered from time to time, having seen their boss do the really dirty work.

• To clean a bathtub properly and thoroughly, one must remove their shoes and get *in* the tub. All tile work, faucet/hardware, and the tub itself should be scrubbed free of mildew, hard water stains, etc. This is assuming that the tub was in at least decent condition before the maid commenced work. If, for example, a shower stall door is covered in water stains because no one has squeegeed in ten years of use… well, don't expect miracles from the maid, because a miracle is what it would take. I've tried all the wretched chemicals made to remove calc and mineral deposits from tile and glass—and they only work to a certain point.

• After the tub, tiles, and/or shower stall have been cleaned, the faucet and hardware should be wiped dry so that they shine.

• Next, the toilet. My method of choice is first to wipe the entire surface with paper towels and throw them away. Then, using the toilet brush, the entire inside of the bowl and the underside of the seat should be scrubbed and the toilet flushed several times to rinse away the cleaning agent and dirt.

Then the top of the seat (to be clear: the place where you sit) is sprayed with a cleaning agent and wiped with paper towels.

Finally, the entire outside, from top of the tank down to the back and bottom where it is fastened to the floor, is thoroughly cleaned and dried.

- The sink should be scrubbed with a sponge, taking care to reach under the rim and around the drain. The hardware should be scrubbed, with attention to the area behind the faucet between the sink and the mirror. This is an area I often check to determine if I am working with a superior or so-so servant. If the sink is clean but the area behind the faucet and handles is gunky and mildewed... we have a talk. All surfaces should be dried.

- Wipe down the counter, clean the mirror, and wipe the face of the cabinets. The door and baseboards should be checked for dirt and dust.

- Place all bathroom items *exactly* where they were.

- The last step is cleaning the floor. First wipe up any water that has pooled from cleaning. Then sweep, mop, and dry.

- As a final and most important touch, a paper towel should be used to trace the entire edge of the bathroom floor and baseboards. No matter what mop is used, mops are too big to finesse the edge of the wall, in the corners and under the edges of the cabinets. One of my "tests" is to go into a "cleaned" bathroom and run a piece of tissue in the corner behind the bathroom door as well as behind the toilet. Maids get a new understanding of clean after watching that, because that 3-second wipe usually yields a dirty, dusty, hairy tissue and a reminder of why I'm the boss. (I've also been on the receiving end of lessons like this. They are useful.)

The bathroom should also be viewed from different angles before leaving. Are there streaks on the mirror? Has a random hair been left behind in the sink or tub? Is the tissue roll full or almost empty and in need of replacement? Does everything sparkle?

Throughout the cleaning, the washer and dryer should be checked, so the maximum number of loads that can be completed during the 3-hour period aren't sitting in the washer for an hour or two, forgotten.

As this is a basic clean, the details of dusting, vacuuming, and folding and putting laundry away are not expected. However, each room should have the large surfaces dusted, throw rugs picked up and shaken *outside,* chairs and light items moved aside for vacuuming, and everything left in a general state of order.

Let's pause to elaborate on the shaking out of rugs. Too many times I've seen a maid grab a throw rug and shake it right there, sending a dust bomb into the room with a plan to vacuum up the mess. She should shake the rugs outside, away from the door, patio furniture, etc. so dirt, hair, and dust cannot fly back onto anything else other than earth or concrete.

If your maids follow this outline, you will receive an excellent and efficient clean that should be scheduled every week or at least every other week, if possible.

Yes, we can all do this work. We might be very good at it and actually enjoy and take pride in it (I do). Some people consider cleaning therapeutic and get a good feeling from making a place shine… but not when raising an infant! Your time needs to be focused on your spouse/partner and baby—not on the hair and dust stuck behind the toilet!

If it's in your budget, schedule 5-hour or all-day cleanings—then you can expect much more. Everyone will require something different, but a few things you can expect with a full-day cleaning include:

- The kitchen will receive a much deeper clean. The inside of the fridge and freezer will be wiped. Multiple loads of dishes and hand washing will be done. Stains on the pots and pans will be scrubbed and removed. (For example, stainless steel pots require serious scrubbing with a product such as Barkeepers Friend from time to time.)

- Dusting will include every knick-knack, the tops and faces of picture frames, baseboards, and detail in carved doors.

- Vacuuming will include removing pillows and cushions from chairs and sofas and using attachments to vacuum the upholstery. The maid will also maintain the vacuum and replace the bag frequently (do not allow a maid to use her vacuum—or any tools for that matter that are used in countless strangers' homes. Buy and supply your own tools).

- Laundry will be folded and put away, bed linens changed, and fresh towels put in the bathrooms and kitchen.

Now that you know what this servant should do, how do you find her and how much does the service cost?

Costs vary greatly across the country. In Silicon Valley, for example, every tech IPO pushes up the cost of everything, so even the weakest of service providers will claim around $20 per hour. In small towns in smaller states, the fee could be half that.

The ideal way to find your maid is to ask a trusted friend or neighbor for a reference. Usually, even though they carefully guard the time they have with their maid (if she is excellent), they will give you her contact information.

When I owned my cleaning business, I told my clients that I did not like to go into "strangers" homes, and that nice people don't like strangers coming in theirs. But friends of friends are always welcome… so I asked them for referrals.

If you can't find a maid that way, you will either have to search online or through an agency (and agency placements will always be much more expensive because there are more hands in the pie).

Whether you require a maid to be licensed, bonded, and insured will be a personal decision. As a maid and the owner of a company with employees, I had all the coverage. Clients found comfort in that. If you hire people without insurance, you're assuming some risks, and know that if anything is broken or goes missing—you pay.

I was incredibly strict in my "replacement" policy. Even if my employees broke the smallest item, I replaced it. For example, I had a client who—I thought neurotically—had dozens and dozens of tiny, blown-glass bottles on the edge of her bathtub. It definitely made for a precarious clean, and I couldn't imagine bathing there. One time, as was inevitable, we broke one of the bottles.

The client laughed and said, "Thank God! I need to get rid of those."

I told her that we must replace it, and that if she wanted to reduce the number of bottles on her bathtub edge, she would have to do it... not through attrition at my maids' hands. She said no. I insisted—then spent the day driving from one side of town to the other, combing knick-knack stores until I found a replacement.

However, it's not advisable to expect this level of service. If you're concerned, be sure to request proof of insurance and other documentation.

Speaking of expectations... as you may have gathered, mine are rather high. However, they are—I believe—fair. If I'm receiving so-so service, that's fine if I'm paying a so-so rate. If I'm receiving superior service, I expect to pay for it. I'm willing to train, write lists and directions, and allow a grace period for the learning curve. Any mistake (anything done intentionally is, obviously, not a mistake) can be made once and forgotten.

A lesson I learned from my cousin who's owned multiple service businesses: if you find someone who can do 80% of what you request, you've got it made. Hold on to that person! Expecting more is a set-up for mutual frustration. If your staff is working below 80%, more training is required. If they are below 60%, like in school, that's flunking.

A nuance of the rule: expect them to do 80% of what you have asked, and expect it to take up to 50% longer than it would take you. If it takes 75% longer, that's a waste of everyone's time—find someone else.

To conclude, here's a list of small details to consider:

• You will never find a servant who thinks and acts exactly like you. However, there should not be incongruence in the relationship. If your household is a nondrinking, nonsmoking, no cursing household, it would be ideal if your servant doesn't chain-smoke and cuss like a sailor. If you're a die-hard vegan and your servant shows up for work smelling like her drive-through bacon breakfast... you get the idea.

No matter how talented the servants are, if their very presence is an irritant, it won't work.

• A servant should be happy to take direction, advice, and adapt to your style and needs. She should have her own set of skills and routines, but she is working for you. She is not to argue or push her routine.

I had a maid working for me who would refuse to acknowledge me when I made requests.

"Do you hear me?"

"Yes."

"Then I would appreciate you acknowledging what I've said."

She replied with something I can't recall word-for-word, but the gist of it was that she didn't need "help" from me. I was shocked to hear such sass from an employee. I decided to clear the air.

"I'm going out on a limb here… but I'd say it's rather apparent from your cleaning skills and your attitude that you've never cleaned a house in your life, and because you went to college, you think you're too good for this."

Her answer was, in so many words: *Yes.*

This situation is easy to resolve: Pay what is owed and politely escort her to the door. If she needs to work and behaves like that, she can work for someone who has no idea what they need or how to clean. May they be happy together.

• Any rudeness or sass, from either side, is unacceptable. Servants are not doormats, and employers are not paying to deal with "tude." Communication should be clear, open, and respectful.

• It is a wonderful treat when you find help with whom you click, with whom you can make polite, if not also deeply meaningful conversation. Whenever I had this, my servants and I learned much from each other, and remained friends afterwards. If you don't find this kind of relationship right away… keep trying! It's possible, and worth the effort.

CHAPTER EIGHT

The Role of a Cook and How to Find One

This chapter is for those who are dedicated to eating quality meals prepared fresh at home, mostly or entirely from scratch. For folks who are happy with frozen, premade meals, take-out, or meals from boxes, a cook or chef is unnecessary.

However, nice meals at home may be important for you for many reasons:

- You're health conscious and want quality, nutrient-rich foods.

- You like food that is fresh and tastes exceptionally pleasing.

- You realize that—adding up the tally at restaurants—it's often less expensive to have someone cook for you at home.

- You simply love eating at home with your family, but don't have the time to cook three meals a day.

While most of us can't remember a time when this was the case, it used to be fairly common in the United States for people to have a cook or chef in their home. It might be the maid or nanny, but sometimes it was a servant whose only job was to prepare meals.

Since few of us have experience with help in the kitchen, let's look at the differences between a cook and a chef. Although definitions vary, here's an easy distinction:

A **cook** is likely to have less experience and would require directions, if not full-on training, to understand and meet your needs. A cook should, however, know how to... well, cook!

Baking a potato, slicing cheese, and boiling eggs—that's not cooking. Your gardener, pool-boy, and 8-year-old should know how to do those things.

Knowing how to cook includes basic knowledge such as:

- Cookware: what kind is used for what purpose, and to how to use the different types on a gas or electric stove and oven.

- The basics of kitchen hygiene, safe food handling and storage.

- Basic ways to clean and prepare the major food groups: grains, legumes, meats, dairy, vegetables, fruits, nuts and seeds, herbs, and condiments.

- A culinary background and a handful of basic dishes they can prepare well from scratch.

A **chef** is far more experienced, would have a deep and broad understanding of all of the above topics and have a highly refined and diverse set of dishes she can prepare. A chef would require—and want—much less direction in the kitchen, and likely prefer to work their magic, then have you come to the dining table and be surprised with what she's created.

Oooh, la la! It would be nice if we could all have a chef!

But people who want and can afford a chef probably already have one. The rest of us, what we're looking for is a cook, and what we'll likely find is not a cook, but a "prep-cook."

Going back to the example of my nanny who is also little bit cook and a tiny bit maid: I started with unfair expectations of her abilities, given her beaming enthusiasm to try. She was willing to try to cook anything—and got an A for effort every time. However, for texture and taste… sometimes a C, sometimes an F. That was discouraging for her and frustrating for me.

We decided to back up. I should have known that, despite intelligence and enthusiasm, she was still a beginner and would need a lot of training. Our setback was my fault.

Nevertheless, we were undeterred. We changed the role to prep-cook. That is the person in the kitchen who stands with the cook or chef, chopping, cleaning, and generally doing as

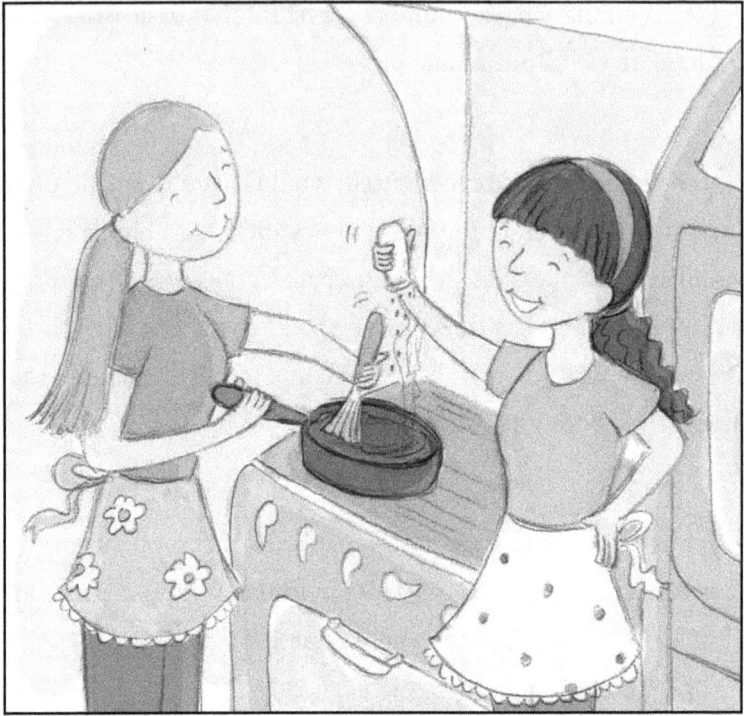

If you are willing to train them, often a nanny will help in different areas. I'm teaching our nanny to cook and we're both having fun in the process.

told, all the while watching the cook and gaining knowledge and experience.

For example, it takes me 48 hours to prepare a pot of soup. The first 24 hours is dedicated to the broth: slow boiling bones with vegetables, herbs, and spices. The prep work for that alone—washing and blanching bones, washing and chopping all the veggies—can take half an hour or more. If there are beans or grains in the soup, I wash them, remove stones and dirt, and soak them overnight. Another half hour. After the broth cooks and cools, I strain it, put in the fridge to cool, and then clean up.

My prep-cook can do all of that very well.

The next day, more veggies must be washed, chopped, and peeled, beans strained, meat—if any—rinsed and browned in flour... you see where we're going here. And that's just the soup!

My cooking style,[5] old-school, takes a long time. Having the help of a prep-cook makes it possible for me to continue to cook and eat this way, even while raising an infant.

Over time, my beloved nanny/prep-cook has become really proficient at several dishes, adds more to her repertoire every day, and with minimal instruction and oversight, can prepare several meals a week.

What a difference that makes! Moms and dads who cook are probably already discussing the idea of a cook with their family members right now... as they should! Just as with cleaning, even if we enjoy cooking, it's hard to enjoy anything when you have to do *everything*, on four hours of sleep a night, for the past six months.

---

5. My cooking style wasn't always like it is now. My understanding of the food pyramid about 25 years ago was: pizza at the bottom as a solid foundation, a healthy variety of drive-through restaurants in the middle, and the top, a small daily bowl of packaged ramen with a "flavor pack."

Whether you hire a separate servant to cook or you have an arrangement with your maid or nanny, having someone to share the cooking duties will help you enjoy your food more, take more pleasure in the time you do spend cooking again, and most importantly, allow you to continue eating well while spending quality time with your baby.

When I advertised for my nanny, I stated what I was looking for in very specific terms. I was not looking for someone to raise my child, rather for someone to help me cook, clean, and care for my baby—*with* me, not *for* me.

It is most efficient and cost-effective to find a nanny or maid and train that person as your prep-cook. Even the busiest maid or nanny will have downtime during her day—time for which she's paid. Prep work in the kitchen is the perfect activity for those time slots.

Whatever you're looking for, as always referrals are best. Short of that, you'll probably be looking online or going through an agency. In any case, the best approach is to state very clearly what you're looking for and what you will pay, ask for your referrals, and go though the hiring process as we've outlined for all other servants.

A final note: I like to set an agreement with all domestic servants that the first week or two is a trial period to determine if both parties are happy with the arrangement. At the end of the trial period, if both of us agree, then the job begins. This way there are no false expectations or strong disappointments on either side if there isn't a click.

CHAPTER NINE

The Role of a Nanny and How to Find One

Few people will spend as much time with your baby as your nanny. It is likely that your nanny will spend many more waking hours with your baby than the baby's father—even if he's home from work as soon as he can be and loves being involved.

Therefore, it is critically important that you find the correct person for the job. Yes, I want multi-mega talent. BUT, the top requirement—so non-negotiable that no qualifications can override it—is that she and my baby must adore each other.

Before starting the interview process, I thought the love between my baby and nanny would build slowly if the match were right. That may be so in most instances, but in my case, I was delighted to be mistaken. I interviewed several people, and liked a few of them. But baby did not respond with anything I could call affection or favor. She was about six months old at the time, so maybe she wouldn't respond to any stranger with exuberance.

Wrong!

The moment our nanny-to-be walked in the door, she ran to my baby and started playing with her. My baby lit up with joy. It was like two old friends finding each other after a long separation. I couldn't believe it… but I knew what to do. I secured her in the position as soon as possible.

I interviewed her, asked how she felt about my approach to the mother/nanny relationship, asked if she were willing to help cook, and confirmed that she understood I would never leave her alone at home with my baby.

Not only did she understand what I was trying to establish, she was also enthusiastic about the unique approach. She admitted she didn't know much about cooking—but said she would love to learn. She even *volunteered* to do the cleaning when I said I was also looking for a part-time maid.

What an attitude!

Further, she had excellent experience with postpartum mothers and their thousand questions: "Is it normal when the baby… My boob looks like… The poo-poo is …" Even questions out of left field: "Hey, we're moving next week—wanna work extra hours and help us pack?"

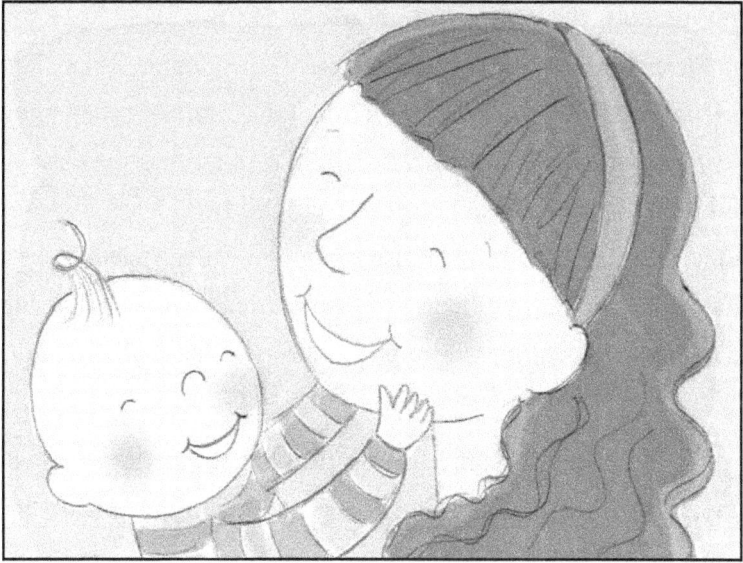

*First and foremost, a nanny should love babies...
especially yours!*

Her experience ranged from newborns to teens, she had excellent presence, a good work ethic, a genuine love of learning, and an intense love for children—especially mine!

She and I send each other text messages on her off-days to discuss my baby's new achievements. We cry together when she does something new or we look at her old baby pictures. We plan our fun-, love-, and learning-filled days *together*.

Nanny, like other servant roles, is one that requires no special training, no license, no certification, nor experience. It only requires the gall to call oneself "a nanny." There are many wonderful nannies and even instances where a nanny is far more qualified and even more loving than the mother. Then there are many mediocre so-so's who get the job done dependably and safely—but don't expect that your child will learn a second language or pick up a musical instrument. Then there are those who should be calling themselves "babysitter"—at best. The title of nanny speaks of greater responsibility and, naturally, suggests higher pay.

Since there is no official definition of babysitter and nanny, how do we distinguish between them and determine what pay is appropriate?

Here is a list of some of the duties and responsibilities I would expect of a **babysitter:**

- Play safe and fun games with the children.

- Guide the children in quiet time with activities such as reading or walks in the garden.

- Reheat and serve food.

- Very basic knowledge of baby care, including diapers, dressing appropriately for different weather, and how to put a child to bed.

- Knowing—and being responsible—to check on a sleeping baby frequently (if not staying in the same room).

- Ability to remain calm and take appropriate steps if a baby is hurt: secure baby, call parents, or call 911.

- Dependability—when accepting a babysitting job, she honors the appointment.

If the only thing your nanny can do beyond that is drive… she still has the title of babysitter in my book.

Many neighborhood kids and I possessed the skills listed above when we were 11 or 12. Back then a strong wage was $2 an hour. Today, depending on the part of the country, a babysitter would earn between $5 and $12 an hour.

Nannies, on the other hand, command much greater pay. On the West Coast, this can mean $15–$30 an hour. If their requested pay range is $15–$20, they will likely receive $20 per hour if they only work a few hours a week. If they work over 20–25 hours a week, or they come every day, the hourly rate should go down—basic "volume discount" pricing that applies in most businesses.

Many women with the skills (or less) of a babysitter call themselves "nanny" because they drive and work full-time— or worse, my least favorite explanation—because they have a college degree.

I know a nanny who receives $17 an hour to play with a five-year-old. They watch TV, they read books, she warms his dinner, and puts him down for a nap or bedtime. That's it. (Clearly, she failed to be inspired by *The Sound of Music*.) I wasn't the first person to ask the mother: *Shouldn't she at least straighten the house while he naps or wash the dishes after he eats?*

The mom responded that she was so happy to find someone whom she trusted that she didn't care if she didn't do anything but sit with her son. If I were going to leave my child alone with someone, perhaps that would be my one and only requirement, too.

Hopefully, the majority of us can hope for more than that from the person we call our nanny. Ideally, the nanny would pride herself in being more helpful and being well rounded in her skills.

In addition to the list above, here are some skills we might require:

• Clean driving record, safe vehicle, and willing to run errands.

• Certified in CPR.

• Some knowledge of food preparation.

• Some knowledge of child development—what communication skills and abilities one can generally expect at what age, and how to best engage children at different stages.

- They don't need to be teachers, but they should take an active interest in your baby's development—reading books, playing educational games, and singing with your baby (trained voice or not. I know first-hand that babies love your singing even if it offends the general public.).

For fun and to teach her to communicate before she began speaking, I'd been teaching my baby sign language since she was born. My nanny was thrilled with that. Though she'd never learned ASL (American Sign Language) before, she picked it up immediately, and practiced it with my baby. The three of us clap and sing every time my baby uses a new sign.

Is it beginning to sound like my nanny is more like a big sister or auntie to my baby? She may as well be, and the three of us are as happy as can be. This, however, is not intended to imply that there is never friction. There are shortcomings, things "goofed," and moments of impatience—from both sides. We work through the issues: I teach her actions and skills she lacks; and she accepts that sleep deprivation is a real phenomenon (a method of torture, in fact) that renders a mom less diplomatic than normal.

- Takes direction *very* well. This skill is a requirement as great or greater than any other. If your maid has a personality similar to, for example, a donkey, sometimes you're going to have items placed and cleaned incorrectly, or just not done the way you requested. Irritating, but no biggie.

If your cook has a donkey personality, you might be served something different than you requested. Well, so what? You'll learn to like her food, her way, or you'll find someone else.

If your nanny insists that her way to [fill in the blank] is better than the way you've requested, your baby is going to be exposed to something you didn't want—and that is unacceptable.

Whether or not the mother knows best, the mother knows best. Her husband can offer advice and set policy with her, her relatives can suggest different ways, and even the nanny can ask if the mother "has considered" this or that.

But in the end, the father generally doesn't raise the newborn—the mother does. The father, relatives, and friends come and go as they please or need. The mother stays with the baby, caring for her every need.

With that understanding, the servant doesn't give orders to the mother regarding how to raise her baby. Servants, and this goes for neighbors, too, don't tell a mother what's best for her baby. Some examples:

We may believe that giving soda to a baby is a form of cruelty, but we do not have the right to tell that to a mother stuffing her baby with carbonated, corn-syrup beverages—unless she asks for our thoughts.

We may believe that it's sad for both mother and baby to choose pharmaceutical formula over breast milk when the only reason is that it frees the mother from caring for the baby—but that's her right.

We may believe that these things cause harm to the child, but since they are common practices, many people choose them. Whether we think this qualifies them for the joy of busting rocks, we must keep it to ourselves.

I happen to believe it's best to make fresh organic food for my children and to disallow junk food. Believe it or not, many people have worked to change my mind, citing my cruelty in not giving my infant artificial colors, GMO white flour, and GMO sugar all baked together in an aluminum pan for her birthday.

Hey, that's my right. It's best to grin and ignore concerns. Remember all the strange comments people made to you while you were pregnant, and how you usually decided to ignore them? Same thing.

My cousin and his wife were pregnant with twins. They were trying to decide on names, and the wife (knowingly) had requested that they not probe family and friends for their opinions. My cousin, on the other hand, wanted name-by-committee. He asked neighbors, colleagues, and passers-by. One day, he came back to the car after buying something in a 7-Eleven and said to his wife,

"Hey, I'm bummed but I think we need to find new names."

"Why?"

"That guy in there really didn't like them."

"What guy?"

"The guy working the cash register."

From there, it got worse: he asked his mother. His mother—her mother-in-law—told them in no uncertain terms, "I can't have grandchildren with those names."

Guess what happened. They got those names.

Running interference is a part of motherhood: grandmas will give your kids garbage to eat; babysitters (if you leave them alone) may allow children to see things on TV you wouldn't tolerate; dad will play more roughly with them when you're not looking, screw-up their schedule, and not remember what or when to feed them.

But stand firm in your right to raise your baby as you see best. The result of the methods we choose is between us and our baby, and though there will be differing opinions in the public, you do not have to tolerate your wishes being undermined by people you're paying to help you, especially your nanny.

As for the mother-in-law, whatever she's doing or saying... get used to it, and if possible, find a way to love her anyway.

As with most relationships in our lives, if we choose the wrong nanny, it can be worse than not having one at all. The good news with the nanny relationship, however, is it's easy to part ways. Keep looking until you find one with whom you feel the super "click."

When I'm out and about during the day with my baby, I usually see many more babies with nannies than with their mothers. In the beginning I assumed these women walking their babies, singing to them, playing with them in the park, and showering them with love were the moms.

Slowly I figured out that it's a better bet that it's the nanny— and to be surprised if it's the mom. I guess I assumed that a lot of people had babies when they were 18–20—or conversely, 45 years old—and that their babies were many different looks and colors than they were! Sometimes I'm a little slow, or maybe I thought that was common because I'm an older mom with a baby whose features are not all from my racial gene pool.

The wonderful news is, though the babies would likely rather be with their mothers, I've observed wonderful interactions between baby and nanny. I've been so happy for the babies, the mothers, and the nannies to see that these babies are being cared for marvelously. I know it's not always the case, but I've seen a lot of exemplary care.

Whether you use a nanny to help you while you are with your baby or while you are away… go to the lengths necessary to find not the "perfect nanny," but the perfect one for you.

Where Do We Go From Here?

As I mentioned in the introduction, I was raised in Texas. In that state, and I guess the entire US of A for that matter, we're still living the legacy of the pioneer settlers, which is:

By golly, if I need something, I can pick myself up by my bootstraps and git it!

I grew up with that mindset. It was the culture and a necessity in my home. I rarely received—and eventually stopped wanting—help. It seemed like a weakness. Shoot, for a long time it was even a little tough to accept love... it seemed a little like help.

As a late friend of mine from Australia said, "America is the land of orphans," meaning that Americans were the most isolated people he'd ever met. We may live on top of each other in physically dense communities, but sit on the porch at sunset with your neighbor every evening? Plant kitchen gardens with the neighborhood children? Live together in love and common goals with relatives and *really* help each other?

We don't help each other and we don't even hire much help. We're still living the pioneer life—but we're not on the prairie with our families anymore. It's time for some adjustments to our approach to our work, in and outside the home, and to the resulting way we spend time (or not) with our families.

A resilient self-sufficiency is fantastic, something we want to continue to have and teach our children. But let's not stop there.

In my early 20's I commenced my mission to travel the world (alone and with my own money, goll-dang-it), and by the end of a decade or so, I'd been to about 50 countries, and had my image of life turned on its head.

I discovered that not all women raced back to work six weeks after childbirth wearing 6" shoulder pads (my travels started in the late '80s), wielding their briefcases, feeding children fast food they wouldn't eat themselves, leaving the care of their families to food factories and daycare—or worse, a TV, and leaving the resulting mental and physical dysfunctions to doctors, pharmaceutical companies, and other industries.

In country after country, I remember seeing mothers rush out to fresh markets as early as possible each morning so the three meals they cooked for their families would have quality ingredients—not the picked-over, wilted remains of the early morning frenzy.

I saw neighborhood women (from all except perhaps the very lowest economic strata) gather during the day for tea while their servants cleaned and assisted them with meal preparation.

I saw mothers keeping their babies with or on them all day and night.

What was most shocking to me was…they looked like they… could it be… *enjoyed* their lives?

They had, of course, their own list of complaints. But overall, I saw women caring for their families, families gathering regularly for home-cooked meals, neighborhood children playing and growing up together in the streets and parks near their homes, and it looked wonderful. It looked healthy and loving!

My first and most pronounced experience with this was in Turkey. A friend of mine knew I was traveling in Europe and offered to introduce me to his extended family in Istanbul. I was 21 years old at the time. When I arrived, the family greeted me at the airport with flowers and shouts of joy and welcome. When I say family, I mean *family*: his parents, aunt, uncle, and cousins— greeting me as a long-lost family member.

They invited me to stay in their vacation home in the south on the Mediterranean. It was only supposed to be for a weekend, but I stayed a month. His aunt Turkan and I adopted each other as mother and daughter. Day and night we ran errands together, shopped for food, cooked, tried to talk (with the 10 words we understood of each other's language), and had a blast.

I couldn't believe the amount of time she spent shopping, preparing food and cooking for her family. I'd never seen anything like it. Their fulltime servant Sultan helped, but Turkan ran the show and worked all day. Her food was astonishingly good: from fish caught that morning, fruit picked only hours earlier, grains grown locally, eggs from a neighbor's yard, and animals we saw hanging at the butcher's, where they'd been slaughtered.

She made breakfast of bread, feta cheese, mountains of fruit, a boiled egg, butter, olives, honey, cherry preserves, and tea.

Lunch and dinner were multi-course feasts of traditional Turkish dishes always followed by dessert of a dozen local fruits.

Mid-afternoon we'd take a break on the front patio, watch the sea, drink tea, and eat a delicious cake or bread she'd baked—then off for an afternoon nap.

See why my two-day stay turned into a month? I'm surprised I ever left.

I've always felt gratitude to Turkan for her loving hospitality and for giving me the gift of knowledge: the knowledge of the joy and beauty in homemaking and motherhood.

I met women leading similar lives all over the world: in Europe, the Middle East, North Africa, Central and South America, and Southeast Asia.

Cynics will say that it's because they can't afford, or don't know any better.

Are those cynics, by chance, the ones trying to introduce

or build yet another megamall in those villages and towns? To convince women that it is more powerful to rush back to their position at work (where they're paid less than a man) than to care for their babies? To sell them plastic diapers, food, and life?

In our "rich" country, we say the women in those other countries can't afford to have the "good life," so they have to stay in tight family units, remain home with their babies, and cook for their families.

But then we say: *We can't afford to stay with our families.* We have to work. We have to have other people raise our babies and feed our families. Here in the U.S., most often it is a choice. We decide what kind of life we want and how much time to spend in the love and care of our families.

For some people, the choice to stay home full-time and affording full-time help is easy. For most of us, choosing to stay home and care for our families will require loss of one income, and sacrifices of our material lifestyle will be required.

For some women, the choice to return to work is simply their desire—even soon after her baby is born. For others, working is legitimately not a choice, as she must return to work.

Whatever the case, most of us can afford to stay home with our babies and raise them, with a little or a lot of help from servants… if that becomes our top priority. I say this with a lot of love and compassion for all moms, including myself. They say being a mother is the toughest job. Working to be a good and present mother most definitely is.

I hope that the information in this book will help mothers get the Help they need to help them realize their dreams of motherhood and family!

For those who feel they can't afford much or any help, or just don't want to hire help for other reasons, there are answers for you, too. It's harder, but there are many ways you can reclaim the care and at least a little more time with your family, which is the subject of my book *Free Love: Everyday Ideas for Joyful Living*.

In *Free Love* you'll find ideas for the kitchen—but not just a few recipes. I offer a completely different approach to work in the kitchen that results in enormous time and money savings, is healthy, fast, EASY, and imagine this… lots of fun, too! There are suggestions for families at any income level, even those with extremely busy schedules, to create a more beautiful, loving, and nurturing home environment—without spending a dime. And finally, my book offers very specific ideas for how today's nuclear families, entirely isolated and alone in raising their children, can begin to rebuild their "village" and enjoy all the joy and support that community offers.

If you've found this book helpful or entertaining, and whether or not you hire help, you will likely enjoy *Free Love*.

In the meantime, if you have comments, feedback, or questions, I'd enjoy hearing from you. You can contact me through my website: www.alliechee.com.

May the long time sun

Shine upon you,

All love surround you,

And the pure light within you

Guide your way on.

- from the tradition of Kundalini Yoga

GIVING BACK

A portion of the proceeds from *New Mother* are donated to **The Isabel Allende Foundation.**

The Isabel Allende Foundation is guided by a vision of a world in which women have achieved social and economic justice.

This vision includes empowerment of women and girls and protection of women and children.

The foundation supports select nonprofits in the San Francisco Bay Area and Chile whose missions are to provide women and girls with:
- Reproductive self-determination
- Healthcare
- Education
- Protection from violence, exploitation and/or discrimination

For more information, visit **www.isabelallendefoundation.org**.

Connect with Allie Chee

Website

www.alliechee.com

Blog

www.alliechee.blogspot.com

Facebook

www.facebook.com/AllieChee

ALSO FROM ALLIE CHEE

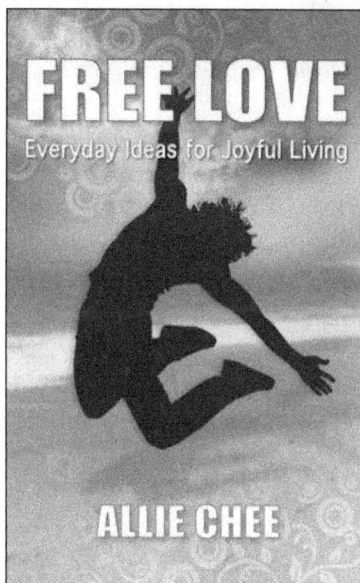

- If you believe family & friends are your greatest treasures
- If you love caring & cooking for them (or want to learn more)
- If you believe that no matter what income, and no matter what schedule demands—friends, family & community can remain our top priorities...

...FREE LOVE was written for you!